THE LONGEVITY SOURCEBOOK

THE LONGEVITY
SOURCEBOOK

BY

DAVID SEIDMAN

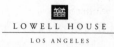

LOWELL HOUSE

LOS ANGELES

CONTEMPORARY BOOKS

CHICAGO

Library of Congress Cataloging in Publication Data

Seidman, David, 1958-
    The longevity sourcebook / by David Seidman.
        p.   cm.
    Includes bibliographical references and index.
    ISBN 1-56565-789-6
    1. Longevity—Popular works.   I. Title.
RA776.75.S44   1997
613' .0438—DC21

97-30843
CIP

Requests for such permissions should be addressed to:
Lowell House
2020 Avenue of the Stars, Suite 300
Los Angeles, CA 90067

Lowell House books can be purchased at special discounts when ordered in bulk for premiums and special sales.

Publisher: Jack Artenstein
Associate Publisher, Lowell House Adult: Bud Sperry
Managing Editor: Maria Magallanes
Text design: Laurie Young

Photo credits: p. 227—SuperStock
all others—courtesy of Bud Sperry and Laurie Young

Manufactured in the United States of America
10 9 8 7 6 5 4 3 2

To the geezers:

Marvin and Phyliss Seidman

Ruth and Marshall Goldberg

Howard and Carol Seedman

Stick around. We need you.

CONTENTS

ACKNOWLEDGMENTS   IX

INTRODUCTION: THE BATTLEFIELD   XIII

PART ONE: THE LONG-LIVED PROFILE   1

How Long Can People Expect to Live?   3
What Will Kill You?   3
Maximum Lifespan   5
Beyond Human Control   7
What Kind of Body Should You Build?   14
What Kind of Mind Should You Have?   18
What Kind of Life Should You Lead?   25

PART TWO: FOOD   27

The Power of Food   29
What's in Your Food?   31
So, What Should You Eat?   89
Buying, Cooking, and Eating   95

PART THREE: EXERCISE   109

Exercise Myths, Legends, and Lies   115
Getting Started   120
Exercise Schedules   123
Specific Exercises   126

PART FOUR: WAYS OF LIVING   155

Training the Mind   157
Control of Your Life   167
Work   172
Sleep   178
Sex   188
Contact with Others   190
Where to Live   199
Smoking   215

PART FIVE: SUPPLEMENTS AND MEDICATIONS   227

Dietary Supplements   231
Glands and Hormones   252
Other Substances   261
Drugs   264

PART SIX: THE FUTURE   271

Theories of Accumulation   273
Theories of Programmed Death   279
Other Theories   281
Is There a Single Answer?   293

AFTERWORD   295
GLOSSARY   297
BIBLIOGRAPHY   305
INDEX   309

ACKNOWLEDGMENTS

Many thanks to the following people:

Madison Lewis, my research assistant: hardworking, dedicated, and patient; my editor, Bud Sperry, who gave me the opportunity to write this book; Michael Hamilburg, who told me to call Bud Sperry; Laurie Young, who designed the book; and Paul Levine, who negotiated the contract.

To the libraries whose holdings made researching the book possible:

Biomedical Library and College Library of the University of California, Los Angeles;
Gerontology Library and Doheny Library of the University of Southern California;
Culver City and West Hollywood branches of the Los Angeles County Library;
Beverly Hills Public Library;
Main branch and Montana Avenue branch of the Santa Monica Public Library;
Brentwood branch of the Los Angeles Public Library; and
Science, Technology, and Patents room of the Los Angeles Central Library.

I owe additional thanks to the friends, relatives, and colleagues who offered encouragement, support, and a willing ear, even if I annoyed them with talk of high-density lipoproteins or the difficulties of book publishing.

Mike Aragona
Cliff Biggers
Kurt Busiek
Stacey and Mark Conchelos
Jackie Estrada
Michele Findler

Nat Gertler
Dave Gibbons
Cheryl Gurin
Pamela Hazelton
Tony Isabella
Mark Lamana
Brian Saner Lamken
Julie Lesser
Allison Littleton
Maria Magallanes
Sadie McFarlane
Michael Avon Oeming
Marilyn Papiewski
Jacquelyn Schnoop
Mark and Mary Seidman
Marvin and Phyliss Seidman
Rod Underhill
Linda and Barry Wehrli
Dr. Marianne Young

Finally, I owe my deepest thanks to the many authors, doctors, researchers, and others who wrote about longevity before I came along. Some of them are mentioned prominently in the text. Others are not, especially if their main value was in confirming the statements of the ones quoted more often. But they were all important:

David Armstrong, Robert Arnot, Louis Aronne, Neil Barnard, Cynthia Beall, Denis Bellamy, Gillian Bentley, Phil Berardelli, Walter M. Bortz II, Jane E. Brody, Sue Browder, Marian Burros, Jean Carper, Deepak Chopra, Winifred Conkling, Geoffrey Cowley, Douglas Crews, Richard Deeb, Vladimir Dilman, Augustine Gaspar DiGiovanna, Doug Dollemore, Peter Doskoch, Wesley Du Charme, Caleb Finch, Norman D. Ford, Michael Fossel, Deborah Franklin, Naomi Freundlich, James Fries, Stanley Garn, Ralph Garruto, Dan Georgakas, Linda Gerber, Mark Giuliucci, Malcolm Gladwell, Robert Goldman, Peter Gorner, Denise Grady, Fred Graver, Katharine Greider, H. Winter Griffith,

Leonard Hayflick, M.S. Kanungo, Solomon Katz, Ronald Klatz, Jeffrey Kluger, Ronald Kotulak, Larry Laudan, Thomas Maugh II, Peter Mayer, John J. Medina, Earl Mindell, Christine Mlot, Tom Monte, Thomas Moore, Carol Orlock, Stephen Rae, Robert Ricklefs, Robert Rosenblatt, David Ryback, Jessica Snyder Sachs, Michael Segell, Gail Sheehy, Rajindar Sohal, William Stini, Robert Stock, Trudy Turner, Lisa Walford, Roy Walford, Stephen Weeks, Richard Weindruch, Kenneth Weiss, Mark Weiss, Mark Williams, Robert Willix, Ruth Winter, James Wood, John D. Young, The Centers for Disease Control, the editors of *Men's Health* magazine, the editors of *Prevention* magazine, the editors of Reader's Digest Books, the editors of Time-Life Books, Metropolitan Life Insurance Company, United States Department of Agriculture, United States Department of Health and Human Services.

They are the real authors of this book.

DAVID SEIDMAN

INTRODUCTION:
THE BATTLEFIELD

IN ANY CROWDED ROOM, SPARK UP A CONVERSATION ABOUT LONGEVITY. Then duck and yell, "Incoming!"

Yoga, someone will claim, is the best way to a long life. Someone else will make the case for tennis or for sex. Alcohol is good for your heart, someone will say. No, another person will declare; alcohol will kill you. Somebody will call meditation the key, while another plumps for selenium capsules and a third speaks out for hormone replacement therapy. Yet another person will say flatly that none of the above matters; your genes are the determining factor.

Even the experts disagree. Authorities and quacks fill the bookstores and talk shows with conflicting theories. The most dignified scientists can fight like prairie bobcats.

And it's been that way ever since people realized that they didn't necessarily have to die young. Longevity theories go back more than 5,000 years, filling scrolls and universities and cocktail parties with wild speculation and fiery argument.

This situation annoys me. Longevity is literally a matter of life and death, so I want clear, straightforward answers.

Hence this book.

The Longevity Sourcebook surveys the experts and compiles the major truths, myths, and opinions on longevity. Where the experts disagree, this book will sort out the arguments on both sides and note how the scientific consensus votes.

As to what I'm doing here: I am a journalist. I've worked for publications from the *Los Angeles Times* (as editor and writer) and the *San Francisco Examiner* to the medical magazine *RX Home Care*. When my editor said that he was interested in a longevity book, I jumped at the chance.

What I'm not is a diet promoter or academic theorist. My job here is to explain and clarify the swarm of information and passionate claims that fill the world of longevity.

Of course, anyone working in longevity eventually hears the sentiment, "If living a long time means giving up the things I like, then I'd rather die young."

I don't object any too strongly to that gripe. If someone wants to take actions that will make him die before I do, I have a simple response: "Be my guest." The rest of us will live a long time, and I hope that this volume will help.

This is a sourcebook, not a prescription pad. If you want to act on any of the ideas in this book, *talk to your doctor first!*

Now, let's go into battle.

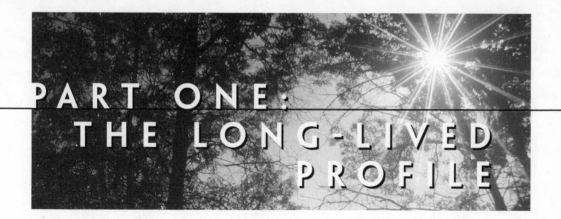

PART ONE:
THE LONG-LIVED
PROFILE

HOW LONG CAN PEOPLE EXPECT TO LIVE?

IN THE DAYS OF ANCIENT GREECE WHEN INFANT MORTALITY WAS HIGH, life expectancy was about age 17. In ancient Rome, about 22. In 1776, under 40. In 1900, about 47.

Today, it's about 76. And tomorrow?

Barring a miracle, life expectancy "will probably rise slowly but steadily . . . reaching as high as age 80 by the year 2050," predicts Augustine Gaspar DiGiovanna of Salisbury State University, author of the gerontology text *Human Aging: Biological Perspectives*. Beyond 2050, life expectancy should hit somewhere from 85 to 100.

In the here and now, one of the most reliable ways to beat the life-expectancy odds is, simply, not to die. Some killers are waiting for you—but you can skid around them.

WHAT WILL KILL YOU?

YOU CAN CHEAT DEATH.

American babies born in 1922 had an average life expectancy of less than 65 years—in other words, death by 1987. The babies who beat the odds and were still alive at age 65 had an average life expectancy in 1987 (according to DiGiovanna) of almost 82 years.

How did they stretch their life expectancy?

They avoided the most common deaths.

The National Center for Health Statistics notes that heart disease is by far the leading cause of death among people aged 65 and older. The next cause is cancer, followed by stroke, chronic obstructive lung disease, pneumonia and influenza, diabetes, accidents, atherosclerosis (thickening of artery walls), kidney diseases, and blood infections. According to *Live Longer, Live Better*, a volume covering a wide spectrum of topics concerning senior citizens, "Life-threatening illnesses . . . account for about 80 percent of all deaths in this country."

Some statistics:

- "If cancer were cured tomorrow, about 3.1 years would be added to the life expectation of a newborn and about 1.9 years to the life expectation of a 65-year-old," says Dr. Leonard Hayflick, professor at the University of California at San Francisco School of Medicine, a pioneer of longevity research and author of the book *How and Why We Age*.

- Eliminating heart disease may add five to nine years to a person's life expectancy. Eliminating all major cardiovascular diseases—heart disease, arteriosclerosis, and cerebrovascular diseases such as stroke—can add at least ten years of extra life. Removing both cardiovascular diseases and cancer would increase life expectation by about 17 years.

- "Eliminating [all] top ten causes of death would increase the life expectancy of people over the age of 65 by about 20 years," says *The American Geriatrics Society's Guide to Aging & Health*.

In fact, says Hayflick, eliminating *all* causes now written on death certificates would result in a life expectancy of well over 100 years.

(Not everyone agrees. The authors of *Live Longer, Live Better* say, "Even big drops in the current diseases of the elderly won't raise life expectancy significantly because other diseases will take their place.")

Without ailments, can people live forever—or at least for centuries? Current scientific thought says that there is an upper limit to human life.

THE PERSIANS DIDN'T GO FAR ENOUGH.

"The ancient Persians, who made much of celebrating birthdays, esti-mated that the longest anyone could live was 80 years," writes science and medicine journalist Carol Orlock in her book *The End of Aging: How Medical Science is Changing Our Concept of Old Age.*

Today, no one disputes that more than a century of life—and, in many cases, active and enjoyable life—is possible. In the United States alone, more than 25,000 people are over 100. (Some estimates put the number over 60,000, and growing.)

But that's nothing compared to some of the stories of long lives.

In 1604, an Irish noble known as the Countess of Desmond died at (so it is written) age 140. A Danish sailor named Christian Drakenberg, who died in 1772, was said to have been more than 145. The Soviet Union claimed that Mukhamed Eizavov, an Azerbaijani farmer, lived more than 147 years. Zaro Agha, a Kurdish Turk who died in 1933, said that he was over 150 years old and that he had met Napoleon. Thomas Parr, an English farmer, was said to have been 152 when he died in 1635. A carnival worker named Charlie Smith, who said that he had been a slave, died in 1979, claiming to be 157. Another carny, Joice Heth, described her life as a slave on George Washington's plantation and declared her age at more than 160. Colombia honored Javier Pereira with a stamp when he reached age 167. A Brit, Henry Jenkins, claimed to have lived 169 years when he died in 1670. In 1973, Shirali Mislimov of Azerbaijan died at, allegedly, 170. Li Chung Yun, a Chinese herb seller, died in 1933, more than 190 years old.

None of the above can match the claims of Nicholas Flamel, an alchemist born about 1330 who was said to have lived at least 430 years, or the Comte de Saint-Germain, who about two centuries ago claimed to have lived a span ranging from 188 years to, incredibly, more than a millennium. And, of course, the Bible says that Adam lived more than 900 years, Noah 950, and Methuselah a whopping 969.

Not one of the above claims, which are among the best-known in the longevity literature, has been proved. Almost all of them have been thoroughly quashed.

But the following claims are almost certainly true.

American Delina Filkins, according to consistent reliable records, lived from May 4, 1815, to December 4, 1928, making her 113 years old. A Japanese fisherman named Shigechiyo Izumi (or Shigecko Isumi, depending on your translation) was nearly 121 years old when he died in 1986. And Frenchwoman Jeanne Calment, who was born in February 1875 and died in August 1997, topped 122 years— "her mind still sharp and her tongue witty," according to the *New York Times*.

So much for the maximum age that people have actually attained. What is the maximum life span—that is, the oldest age that the human body can possibly attain?

Most longevity authorities put the maximum life span between 110 and 120 years, although exceptional individuals like Calment and Izumi can slightly exceed that maximum. Other experts go further, quite a few going as high as 130, with a few scattered researchers plumping for 140, 150, or 200.

Standing on the far shores of longevity theory, biology professor Robert Ricklefs at the University of Pennsylvania and Caleb Finch, professor in the neurobiology of aging at the University of Southern California, authors of the book *Aging: A Natural History*, declare that if humanity can wipe out the effects of aging, "50 percent of us would reach the seemingly astonishing age of 1,200 years."

Dr. Vladimir Dilman agrees. Professor of environmental medicine at New York University Medical Center, former head of endocrinology at the Petrov Institute of Oncology in St. Petersburg, and author of the longevity text *Development, Aging, and Disease*, Dilman calls an upper limit on human longevity a myth. If science can find a way to give people of all ages the health and strength that they enjoy at age 30, he says, "this would lead to an increase in the maximal life span to 1,246 years."

Michigan State University professor of clinical medicine Michael Fossel, in his book *Reversing Human Aging*, goes furthest of all: "If we . . . bring your trauma risk back to that of a 39-year-old, your average life span would be 1,777 years"—nearly twice the life of Methuselah.

Do we have to die at all? No one is entirely certain, simply because science has not entirely nailed down why we age and die in the first place. The theories behind longevity and death are covered in this book's final section.

In the meantime, most of us would be happy to make it to a century. Although most of this book shows the pathways to reaching that goal, it's worth a detour to look at the genes and other items that are built into us before we even start on the journey.

BEYOND HUMAN CONTROL

HEREDITY OR ENVIRONMENT? NATURE OR NURTURE? GENETICS OR DIET and exercise?

Both.

First, there's no doubt that long-lived families produce long-lived children.

- Says gerontologist Denis Bellamy, emeritus professor at the University of Wales and author of *Ageing: A Biomedical Perspective*, "Genetic factors predetermine the potential maximum span of life for every species, and, to a greater or lesser extent, the actual length of life for individuals within the species."

- M. S. Kanungo of India's Banaras Hindu University and Institute of Life Sciences agrees. In his book *Genes and Aging,* he says, "the offspring of long-lived parents have longer-than-average life spans."

- "When both parents survive to age 70 or older, the likelihood that their children will reach 90 or 100 is almost twice as great as that found for the general population," Hayflick says. "Clearly, having long-lived parents and grandparents increases the likelihood of achieving great longevity, although it is no guarantee."

But heredity's powers are limited. "Having two parents who survived into their eighties adds only about three years to a child's life expectancy," says Dr. Deepak Chopra, who has been a professor at Tufts University and Boston University School of Medicine, chief of staff at New England Memorial Hospital, and author of the longevity book *Ageless Body, Timeless Mind.* He adds, "No centenarian has ever been recorded who had a centenarian father or mother."

Experts from Dr. John Rowe (director of the MacArthur Foundation Network on Successful Aging) to Dr. Walter M. Bortz II (a Stanford University Medical School professor, past president of the American Geriatrics Society, and author of the books *Dare to Be 100* and *We Live Too Short and Die Too Long*) calculate that genes determine less than a third of the factors involved in life span.

And maybe much less. In the longevity anthology *Biological Anthropology and Aging: Perspectives on Human Variation over the Life Span,* anthropologists Trudy Turner of the University of Wisconsin at Milwaukee and Mark Weiss of Wayne State University write, "If longevity in humans has any inherited component, it is very small." And in his longevity book *The Methuselah Factors: Learning from the World's Longest Living People,* health researcher Dan Georgakas says flatly, "To date, no genetic factor that positively promotes long life has been discovered."

Not yet, that is.

LONGEVITY GENES

"It is likely there are longevity genes," says health reporter Thomas Moore, a fellow at the Center for Health Policy Research at George Washington University, in his book *Life span: Who Lives Longer and Why*. Dr. Robert Arking of Wayne State University has conducted experiments on fruit flies that may indicate the existence of such genes, according to *Live Longer, Live Better: Adding Years to Your Life and Life to Your Years*, by the editors of the Reader's Digest Association.

In bugs or humans, longevity genes probably "act like switches to control chemical reactions," says Hayflick. Such genes may belong to Helen Borley.

Borley, a retired State Department employee, inherited from her long-lived parents a startlingly low level of LDL ("bad" cholesterol) and high HDL ("good" cholesterol)—a combination that can prevent hardening of the arteries and other cardiovascular diseases. The National Heart, Lung, and Blood Institute in Bethesda, Maryland, has been studying Borley's blood samples to find the gene or genes that have given her such an advantage.

KILLER GENES

Whether or not genes can lengthen your life, they can definitely help to shorten it.

- Heart surgeon Robert Willix, author of *Healthy at 100* and the monthly newsletter *Health & Longevity*, says, "Genetic diseases, such as sickle-cell anemia and cystic fibrosis . . . clearly are the results of mismatched or defective genes."

- According to Dr. Neal Barnard, president of the Physicians' Committee for Responsible Aging and author (with cooking and nutrition instructor Jennifer Raymond) of the diet-based longevity book *Eat Right, Live Longer*, for 5 percent of the people with high cholesterol levels (an important risk factor in heart disease), genetics is at fault.

- Genes can encourage cancer, too. About 5 percent of the cases of breast cancer are caused solely by heredity.

   Five percent isn't much. Genes are likelier to carry the likelihood of a disease than to carry the disease itself.

- Willix says that if your father died of a heart attack, you won't necessarily die the same way; but an attack, fatal or not, is likely.

- In *Biological Anthropology,* cardiologist Linda Gerber of Cornell Medical Center and anthropologist Douglas Crews of Ohio State University have written that some people are born predisposed to high blood pressure.

- Moore agrees that genes can encourage high blood pressure, as well as colon cancer and lung cancer.

Fortunately, a genetic predisposition is not a death sentence. You can stretch many of your built-in limits.

CHANGING THE RULES

Take the ability to push blood through the body. Willix maintains that everyone, even people born with weak cardiovascular systems, can increase their cardiovascular capacity through exercise. Barnard notes that while some people naturally build up an amino acid called homocysteine, which can encourage artery blockages, foods rich in B vitamins—fruits and vegetables especially—can lighten the problem. And, according to Bellamy, even people with a tendency toward arteriosclerosis (hardening of the arteries) can improve their chances by "changing diet, reducing cigarette smoking, and treating hypertension [high blood pressure]."

Georgakas says, "The genetic code determines the outer limit for any given individual's development, while the quality of the environment [including the individual's actions] determines how much of the potential capacity is actually realized."

Or as Fossel puts it in *Reversing Human Aging*, "All you have to do [to live longer] is wear your seat belt, exercise, eat carefully (and less), take antioxidant vitamins, avoid smoking, and not antagonize people who carry weapons"—advice that can extend life no matter what your genetic heritage.

GENETIC FACTORS: SEX

Women outlive men.

- Female life expectancy in the United States is over 78 years, while it's under 73 for men.

- Hayflick says that in 1990, "for persons 85 and older, [there were] 259 women for every 100 men" The *New York Times* adds that in 1997, "for every 100 women over 65, there are only 77 men."

- Chopra notes, "80 percent of all centenarians are women."

- And as noted earlier, the only person known without a doubt to live more than 122 years was a woman: France's Jeanne Calment.

This hasn't always been the case. Women throughout most of history have averaged a shorter life than men—largely, but perhaps not entirely, because many women died in childbirth.

But if death by childbirth is eliminated, women may have a greater chance of longer life than men. "Greater female longevity seems to occur in most animal species," says Hayflick (although, he adds, "it is by no means universal").

In humans, the female hormone estrogen can help to prevent artery disease, according to an article in *Biological Anthropology* by Peter Mayer of the State University of New York's Health Science Center at Brooklyn. Mayer adds that women seem to be more immune to infectious diseases such as flu and pneumonia, and to cancers such as leukemia and lymphoma.

On the other hand, many women outlive men for reasons that may have little or nothing to do with genetic or gender-linked factors like estrogen.

According to a 1993 National Center for Health Statistics survey of the most common causes of death, men are 2.39 times more likely than women to suffer fatal auto accidents, 3.84 times more likely to face homicide or "legal intervention" (the criminal justice system), 4.37 times more likely to commit suicide, and 7.44 times more likely to contract HIV (the virus that causes AIDS).

So do women live longer than men because of their genes, their way of life, or other factors?

"The short, but correct, answer," Hayflick says, "is that we do not know with certainty." The jury is still out, and research continues.

GENETIC FACTORS: RACE

Race matters. "The white population has a higher [life expectancy] at birth than does the black population," DiGiovanna says.

According to Hayflick, the average white baby girl born in 1989 has a life expectancy of 79.2 years, but an African American girl only 73.5; a white boy may expect to live 72.7 years, but a black boy only 64.8.

Is the difference genetic or environmental? To put it more clearly, do the genes of African Americans force them to die younger than whites do, or can blacks live as long as whites—or longer?

You don't have to be a statistician to see that a greater proportion of African Americans live in dangerous neighborhoods than whites do. It's not yet clear whether, all things being equal, blacks might generally outlive whites.

Moreover, statistics are scarce on people of mixed race, as well as on people who are neither black nor white, such as Asians and Latinos.

Race matters—but how much and why is not yet clear.

HOW YOU ARE BORN

How old was your mother when you were born?

The children of older mothers don't live as long, on average, as the children of younger mothers, according to studies that Bellamy conducted. He adds that a firstborn child will tend to outlive his later-born siblings, possibly because their mother was younger when she gave birth to the first of her kids.

Why do the children of young mothers have an advantage? One reason is that older mothers bear a larger proportion of stillbirths, premature births, and other troubled newborns than younger mothers. A 47-year-old mother is three times as likely to have a defective birth than a 22-year-old mother, according to Bellamy.

But later-born children who emerge strong and healthy may live long. *Chicago Tribune* reporters Ronald Kotulak and Peter Gorner, authors of *Aging On Hold: Secrets of Living Younger Longer*, report on experiments that the University of California at Irvine's Michael Rose has conducted on fruit flies. Rose has forced the flies to reproduce much later in life than fruit flies usually do. The offspring of these "old parents" live twice as long as ordinary fruit flies. Journalist Malcolm Gladwell has written that in doing so, Rose "has created a race of fruit-fly Methuselahs."

No one knows yet if this practice can work on other animals—including humans—but it remains intriguing.

WHAT NOW?

Most experts believe that living for millennia isn't currently possible. But topping a century is. What's more, people can do it even if their genes might indicate otherwise. "Seventy percent of illness and death is attributable to behaviors that are yours to direct," Bortz says.

The next sections of this book delve into the areas within human control.

WHAT KIND
OF BODY
SHOULD YOU BUILD?

EVERYONE'S HEARD OF AN ELDERLY ATHLETE WHO HAS THE BODY OF A teenager. And everyone's seen people who eat, drink, and smoke too much, never exercise, and live a stressful depressing life in a polluted unhealthy environment: they look 60 years old when they're actually 40.

These differences aren't just a matter of appearance. They indicate how long you're likely to live—and you can alter them.

While chronological or actual age (the amount of time that a person has been alive) increases every second no matter what, biological or vital age (how well the body looks and functions) is more flexible. "The difference between your vital and your actual age can be as much as 30 years," says Stanford University medical professor James Fries in his book *Living Well: Taking Care of Your Health in the Middle and Later Years*.

As Robert Ricklefs and Caleb Finch write in *Aging: A Natural History*, "If not for [biological aging], 95 percent of us would celebrate our centenaries."

THE BIOLOGICALLY YOUNG BODY

Slim people generally live longer than heavy people. "The insurance data show that the longest life expectancy is observed at weights that are 5 to 15 percent below average," writes Moore in *Life span*.

Norman Ford, a health journalist and author of *18 Natural Ways to Look and Feel Half Your Age*, explains, "A man or woman who has gained 10 to 15 pounds since age 21, or whose waistline has increased more than two or three inches, has a significantly higher risk of being hit by heart disease, stroke, hypertension, diabetes, cancer, osteoarthritis, gallstones, sleep apnea, pulmonary disease, hormone imbalance, immune system suppression, or blood fat abnormality than a person of normal weight."

IDEAL WEIGHT

Figuring the ideal weight for longevity is a tricky thing. The federal government, the Metropolitan Life Insurance Company, several individual researchers, and the long-running, well-respected program called the Baltimore Longitudinal Study of Aging offer different figures.

Table 1.1 is a chart of the entire ranges of weight, including the lowest and highest weights quoted by almost any authority (even if other authorities don't go that low). A young small-framed person should lean toward the slimmer end of the poundage, and an older and larger person can edge closer to the heavier side.

TABLE 1.1   ENTIRE RANGES OF WEIGHT

MEN		WOMEN	
5'2	106–163	5'	90–137
5'3	112–168	5'1	95–140
5'4	117–173	5'2	99–143
5'5	122–179	5'3	104–147
5'6	128–184	5'4	108–151
5'7	133–190	5'5	113–155
5'8	139–196	5'6	117–159
5'9	144–201	5'7	122–163
5'10	149–207	5'8	126–167
5'11	152–213	5'9	128–170
6'	160–219	5'10	130–173
6'1	166–225	5'11	132–176
6'2	171–232	6'	134–179
6'3	176–238		
6'4	182–244		

Since the range of weights is so wide (more than 60 pounds in some cases), it may help to cut out the extremes—the biggest and smallest numbers quoted by any single authority—and look at the figures that most authorities hold in common (see Table 1.2). Again, a young small-boned person should weigh on the light side of these tables, and an older and bigger person can go to the weightier end.

TABLE 1.2   IDEAL WEIGHT RANGES

MEN			WOMEN	
5'2	128–130		5'	97–100
5'3	130–136		5'1	106–116
5'4	132–143		5'2	108–121
5'5	134–150		5'3	111–127
5'6	136–156		5'4	114–132
5'7	138–163		5'5	117–138
5'8	140–169		5'6	120–143
5'9	144–176		5'7	123–149
5'10	149–180		5'8	126–154
5'11	155–184		5'9	131–160
6'	160–186		5'10	135–165
6'1	166–192		5'11	140–171
6'2	171–197		6'	144–176
6'3	176–202			
6'4	182–207			

STABLE WEIGHT

If your body doesn't fit within these ranges—especially if it's too heavy—you should consider changing your weight. The sections of this book on food and exercise will give recommendations on life-extending ways to do it.

But check with a doctor before going on a diet or muscle-building program. Fast radical weight gains or losses can shorten your life.

Chopra quotes a study of 11,700 Harvard graduates. "Data collected between 1962 and 1988 revealed that gaining or losing even a moderate amount of weight over a long period of time raised one's risk of mortality . . . including 75 percent higher risk of dying from a heart attack."

One reason, writes University of Arizona anthropologist William Stini in *Biological Anthropology*, is that "repeated weight-gain and weight-loss cycles have the potential of redistributing body fat in the direction of the trunk." He explains, "Fat deposits on the trunk, a pattern most commonly seen in males, relate to risk factors for cardiovascular disease and diabetes to a much greater extent than limb fat deposits or subcutaneous fat."

So even if you're slightly overweight, it may be better to stay at your current weight than to risk yo-yo dieting, which will lead to a bigger gut and a higher risk of heart attack.

Besides, fixating on fat can lead to anxiety and other emotional difficulties, which are life-shortening in themselves, as the next chapter explains.

WHAT KIND OF MIND SHOULD YOU HAVE?

ATTRIBUTES TO HAVE

The literature on longevity reveals that long-lived people are optimistic, active, and resilient. They enjoy life and don't let troubles make them depressed, passive, or inflexible.

According to a study by the University of Georgia Gerontology Center in Athens, reported by journalist Robert Stock in the *New York*

Times, "Centenarians possess an uncanny ability to handle stress . . . to snap back from losses (the deaths of family and friends) that would devastate other people . . . [and] to cope with everyday frustrations."

"That's not to say that you can smoke like a chimney, drink like a fish, eat like a pig, and just psych your sofa-slugging self into being the George Burns of your block," say the authors of *Age Erasers for Women,* a comprehensive volume from the health publisher Rodale Press, and the companion volume, *Age Erasers for Men.* "You have to practice a healthy life-style to avoid most of the conditions that cause us to look and feel old."

But emotions do affect the body.

- *Staying Young: How to Prevent, Slow, or Reverse More than 60 Signs of Aging,* by Tom Monte and the editors of *Prevention* magazine, refers to a study of "35 years' worth of data on the health and psychological status of 200 men who graduated from Harvard University." Dr. Martin Seligman of the University of Pennsylvania studied the data. "The pessimistic men started to come down with the diseases of middle age earlier and more severely than did the optimistic men," he concluded.

- Researchers from Yale University, the University of Pennsylvania, and Australia's Prince of Wales Hospital found that pessimists had greater amounts of T-suppressor cells, which hinder the cells that keep immunity high.

- The Centers for Disease Control has concluded that people who have pessimistic despairing attitudes are likelier to develop heart disease than will optimistic people.

- Breast cancer spreads fastest among women who bottle up—and, presumably, never purge—their negative emotions, according to a 1987 Yale University study.

- Type A personalities—driven, competitive, always rushing, easily angered—often suffer from high blood pressure, high cholesterol, and irregular heartbeat, and are prone to blood-vessel blockages and heart attacks. In fact, Georgakas calls the Type A "the antithesis of a longevous personality."

- The Center for Gerontology and Health Care Research at Brown University asked more than 1,000 older men and women about aging and their day-to-day living. Some believed that the problems in their lives arose from conditions that could be identified and changed; others blamed their problems on aging itself, and therefore felt that their problems couldn't be improved. Over the next four years, the optimists had a death rate 16 percent lower than that of the pessimists.

"Some patients with an optimistic outlook get better even when the therapy is known to be ineffective or even an outright sham," says Moore. He's speaking specifically about high blood pressure, but the principle applies to all kinds of health problems.

How do good feelings work? The authors of *Age Erasers for Men* describe the process: "Optimists may choose healthier life-styles and take more advantage of social supports such as family and friendship. And optimistic men are more likely to feel that they can take charge of their health and not just passively slide down the path toward old age. . . . So optimists are more likely to live longer and age more gently."

But when you feel anxious, depressed, bored, or lonely, you're likely to eat unhealthily, says Robert Aronne, M.D., a professor at Cornell University Medical College, a member of the Laboratory of Human Behavior and Metabolism at Rockefeller University, and the author (with Fred Graver) of *Weigh Less, Live Longer.*

For a guide toward achieving a longevity-oriented personality, see the section of this book on ways of living.

STRESS

Of all the problems of negative feelings, "the greatest threat to long life is stress," writes David Ryback, Ph.D., associate editor of the *Journal of Humanistic Psychology*, in his book *Look 10 Years Younger, Live 10 Years Longer: A Man's Guide*.

Moore explains, "Stress is a term that describes the signals that the biological and social systems send to demand action—or to enable an individual to take action to adjust to a specific environment." Chopra calls the symptoms of stress "signs from the body that it is exceeding its own coping mechanisms."

"Anything—pleasant or unpleasant—that disturbs the equilibrium (sense of balance) of the body or the mind can be defined as a stressor [source of stress]," writes Robert D. Willix Jr., M.D., a charter member of the American Medical Society for Sports Medicine and a fellow of the American College of Sports Medicine, in his book *Healthy at 100: 7 Steps to a Century of Great Health*. Among the most powerful stressors are the death of a spouse, a divorce, or being fired from work.

The damage that stress does comes in many forms.

- "People who report getting angry often in everyday life situations have higher death rates from coronary artery blockage," says Redford Williams, M.D., of Duke University's Behavioral Medicine Research Center (as quoted in *Good Housekeeping* magazine).

- Men who are subject to frequent high stress are seven times likelier than nonstressed men to develop coronary heart diseases, two to three times likelier to suffer a heart attack, and more than four times likelier to die suddenly from heart trouble, say Orlock and Ryback. The levels of blood pressure, fat, and cholesterol in such highly stressed men are higher, report Ryback and the authors of the *Age Erasers* books.

- Douglas LaBier—author of *Modern Madness: The Hidden Link Between Work and Emotional Conflict*—notes that stress at work "causes an estimated 70 to 90 percent of all illnesses," says journalist Sue Browder.

- "Stress has been shown to weaken the immune system and to have an adverse effect on both hormone and cholesterol levels," reports *Staying Young*.

- Stress also causes or is otherwise connected to:

aches in the back, legs, head, and neck	upset stomach
	colitis
swelling of the prostate gland	ulcers
immune system deficiencies	fatigue
impaired mental function	dementia
hormone imbalances	depression
lack of sexual desire	osteoporosis
excess cholesterol	memory loss
loss of appetite	sleeplessness

Not all of these conditions are fatal, but none are conducive to long life. "One study showed that a remarkable 85 percent of all visits to primary-care physicians are for stress-related illnesses," says Willix.

Not everyone agrees that stress is a killer. "The question of the role of stress in longevity still remains open," says Hayflick, noting "the life expectancy of recent presidents is not much different from [that of] men in the general population." (Presidents and other executives, though, may have advantages over people in subordinate jobs. See the section of this book on work for details.)

GOOD STRESS

Not all stress is killing. "Some stress is actually good," Willix says. "Without some stress as stimulation, life would be pretty dull," say the authors of *Live Longer, Live Better*. "Deadlines at work may be just your cup of tea—they get your adrenaline going and make you work better than ever." "Stress can boost your energy, especially if you regard your [stress-producing] task as a challenge and an opportunity," say the authors of *Staying Young*.

Good stress can even extend life. "Stress, the enjoyable kind, can be healthy, as in sexual excitement, social excitement, or physical challenge. In that sense, you *want* to stay stressed as you grow older," says Ryback. In the words of Marilyn Albert, M.D., of Harvard Medical School, who has researched ways to keep an aging brain at its best, "It's not a mater of whether you experience stress or not. It's your attitude toward it."

The difference between good and bad stress is control, with predictability running a close second. If you feel that the forces around you are uncontrollable and unpredictable, you're almost guaranteed to feel stressed. As Barnard puts it, "If an avalanche of work is dumped in your lap, your stress level is likely to be higher than if you are voluntarily tackling a huge challenge."

Techniques for management, reduction, and control of stress are covered later in this book.

INTELLIGENCE AND EDUCATION

Brains are good for longevity. "In general, people with higher intelligence," DiGiovanna says, "tend to live longer."

HOW IT WORKS

Chopra points out, "Above-average intelligence makes it easier for a person to remain in good health, to earn a stable income, and to learn to resolve personal problems. At the other extreme, people with low intelligence often cannot take advantage of books and articles about health and nutrition; they more easily fall into low-income groups that cannot afford good housing, food, and health care."

Some examples:

- Georgakas says, "Statistics show that for white American males who were 22 years of age in 1900, a seven-year advantage in average life span was enjoyed by those who graduated with honors from universities, and for most of this century, among white males, college graduates have usually outlived the eighth-grade dropouts by an average of five years."

- A U.S. government survey, the *Mortality Study of One Million*, examined a habit that's a nearly sure way to early death: smoking. Of the people who didn't complete high school, 45 percent smoked; but among those who had post-college education, just 15 percent smoked.

- Ricklefs and Finch report in *Aging: A Natural History*, "Six studies of different populations in Asia, North America, and Europe have found that higher education protects against dementia in later ages, whereas the lack of education above an eighth-grade equivalent increases the risk." (Although Alzheimer's disease and other forms of dementia are not fatal in themselves, they can lead to sedentary or stressful living, which can shorten life.)

- Georgakas notes that intelligence and education can often lead to "the self-esteem, flexibility, independence, and planning ability so marked in longevous persons." Moore adds, "It is also possible those with more education and [mental] ability are taking conscious steps to prolong their lives, taking actions seen less frequently among those with less education."

ON THE OTHER HAND

"The majority of American centenarians," Hayflick says, "have less than a ninth-grade education."

If the authorities promoting education as a longevity aid are right, how can Hayflick's centenarians live so long? One answer may be that while Hayflick's centenarians may not have much formal education, they may have stretched their minds in other ways.

Information on ways to increase your intelligence and education is available in part four of this book.

WHAT KIND OF LIFE SHOULD YOU LEAD?

STAYING ACTIVE

More than a millennium ago, the religion of Taoism arose in China. In *Search for Immortality*, editors and writers from Time-Life Books report, "Taoist lore was . . . replete with tales of *xian*, humans who practiced yoga and alchemy to achieve immortality."

"[Taoist] monks combined breathing techniques, dietary principles, specific medicines, regular gymnastics, and spiritual exercises with a sexual discipline . . . culminating in an immortal physical body," says Georgakas.

And so arose the idea of using activity to live a long time.

Longevity being as important as it is, other people had their own ideas about actions that keep people alive. One of the most famous of these thinkers was Renaissance noble Luigi Cornaro.

In Cornaro's time, most people didn't live past age 40. But at 83, Cornaro was still alive and productive; in fact, he published a best-seller on longevity.

Cornaro ate sparingly and abjured the sins of the flesh, but even as a very old man, he rode horses, took close care of his estate, and continued to write. Depending on which research you take as genuine, Cornaro lived until he was somewhere from 98 to 103 years old.

From Taoism to Cornaro to George Burns, staying active and avoiding idleness have been keys to longevity.

- Bellamy lists sedentary living and poor social networks alongside high blood pressure and cigarette smoking as signs of the development of fatal coronary heart disease.

- In *Biological Anthropology*, Douglas Crews and Linda Gerber write, "Low levels of habitual physical activity . . . lead to obesity, hypertension, and hypercholesterolemia [high cholesterol levels]."

- "People who enjoy close personal relationships, have many interests, and stay in control of their lives tend to be healthier and to live longer," write the authors of *Live Longer, Live Better*. Georgakas, who has reported on the longevity-promoting power of activities ranging from working at a satisfying career to maintaining contact with friends and family, calls this common pattern "the activist longevity profile."

OVERDOING IT

If activity is good, can too much activity be too much of a good thing?

Over-exercising has its dangers, but in general, says Ford, "The plain fact is that people don't wear out through years of activity. They rust away as soon as they put their feet up and begin to take life easy."

Now what? For specifics on the activities that are the most life-extending, see the sections of this book on exercise and ways of living.

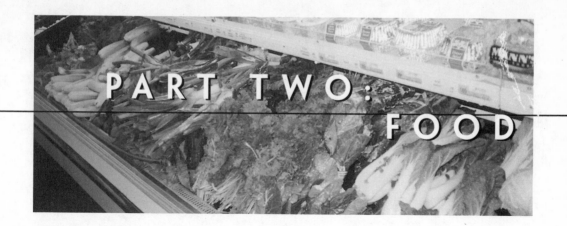

PART TWO: FOOD

*The Lord God planted a garden eastward, in Eden, and there He
put the man whom He had formed. And out of the ground made
the Lord God to grow . . . the tree of life also in the midst of the
garden." But when Adam ate of the tree of knowledge, "the Lord
God said . . . 'Now, lest [the man] put forth his hand, and take
also of the tree of life, and live for ever,' the Lord God sent him
forth from the Garden of Eden.*

GEN. 2:8–3:23

NO THEORY OF LONG LIFE IS MORE COMMON THAN THAT OF A MAGICAL
food, whether from the tree of life or another source. According to Hindu
myth, the northern Indian race called the Utturakuru ate the fruit of a
magic tree and lived for centuries. In medieval times, some Chinese sages
believed that peaches could extend life. The Indians of pre-Columbian
Mexico believed in a life-stretching plant called *octli*.

The Hindus have long spoken of *soma*, an elixir made from plants,
which is said to turn an old body into a young one. They also recommended drinking "viper waters," a mysterious brew that would extend life
for centuries.

The Greek gods were reputed to have drunk ambrosia and nectar to
stay immortal. Around 400 B.C., the Greek historian Herodotus reported
a magical spring in Ethiopia whose waters could rejuvenate anyone who
drank them.

Nineteen centuries later, in 1498, one Marcilio Ficino recommended
drinking the milk of a virgin girl straight from her breast. (The prescription had no medical validity, but the old men who tried it probably didn't
complain.) In the early 1500s, the pioneering alchemist-physician
Paracelsus recommended a probably lethal and definitely disgusting

potion of gold, salt, wine, and horse dung. In the 20th century, experts have touted orange juice, alcohol, garlic, carrots, broccoli, tomatoes, soybeans, rice, and plain old water.

To this day, longevity experts cite food more often than any other factor in life extension. Food can raise—or lower—the likelihood of contracting killers ranging from arteriosclerosis to cancer to diabetes. "The genes that safeguard youth can be controlled by what we eat," say the authors of *Aging on Hold*. The amount of food that you consume, the kinds of foods, the ways that they're prepared, and even the number of meals per day influence longevity.

Before you dig into the details, keep in mind that although the experts quoted in the next sections will make recommendations, not all of them apply equally to everyone.

- In *Ageless Body, Timeless Mind,* Tufts University's Chopra observes, "Centenarians eat a wide variety of diets."

- Dan Georgakas states in *The Methuselah Factors,* "No single diet can ever be designed to meet the needs of all people."

- William Stini, Ph.D., points out in *Biological Anthropology,* "The older a person becomes, the more marked is his or her individuality. Nowhere is this more true than in the area of nutritional needs. Consequently, blanket recommendations for people over 50, 60, 70, or 80 years of age become progressively more error prone."

Nevertheless, Georgakas says, "Despite these wide variations in individual needs, the lifelong eating habits of the longevous contain some constants applicable to everyone."

A good place to start is at the most basic level: the most common ingredients and elements in food.

CALORIES

"Burn your calorie chart," writes Barnard in *Eat Right, Live Longer*.
"There is no need to count calories or to measure portion sizes."

Barnard's view is an extreme one, but many experts share a part of
it—the idea that the amount of calories that you eat is not terribly important in itself.

What matters is the *source* of the calories.

Barnard notes, for example, that "calories coming from potatoes, rice,
pasta, or other high-carbohydrate foods do not have the same effect as
the very same number of calories from chicken, beef, or salad dressing.
The high-carbohydrate foods have much less of a tendency to promote
weight gain."

How does this process work?

Calories are a measure of heat—or at least the amount of potential
heat that foods contain. The body burns calories as a car's engine burns
fuel. If you have too little fuel, you're undernourished. Have too much,
without enough exercise (without running the engine, so to speak) to
burn it off, and your body will have to put the extra calories somewhere.
It stores them in body fat, which is, generally, not great for longevity.

And as Barnard implies, the body burns the calories from carbohydrates more efficiently than it burns calories from fatty foods. You can eat
the same amount of calories in both carbs and fats, but you'll gain less
weight from the carbs.

An exception to this advice is offered by Jean Carper, a journalist who
has written about health for CNN, *USA Weekend*, and King Features
Syndicate. Although she agrees with the other experts that no one should
eat much fat, she believes in keeping all calories, fat or not, to a minimum:
"Eat only enough calories for proper growth and optimum nutrition."

Carper seems to be in the minority, although that minority has some intriguing things to say. For more information, see the following sections on fat, carbohydrates, and caloric restriction.

FAT

Here is some bad news for people who like ice cream and hamburgers: if you want to live a long time, keep away from fat.

Why?

For one thing, long-lived people do it. In his book *The Methuselah Factors*, Georgakas refers to a study of long-lived citizens of the Soviet Union that found that their diets were low in fat. "The diet of the longevous," says Georgakas, "contains about 10 to 15 percent fats"—as well as 10 to 15 percent proteins and 70 to 80 percent carbohydrates. (The typical American, on the other hand, gets close to 40 percent of his calories from fat.)

There is no clear consensus on how much fat is enough. Some experts recommend that it constitute 10 percent of the diet; others allow 25 percent or even 30 percent. But all of them recommend keeping it low.

Why is fat consumption so bad? According to the experts, it can promote:

- heart and circulatory ailments, including high blood pressure, atherosclerosis and coronary artery disease;

- cancers of the lung, prostate, breast, uterus, and colon;

- diabetes;

- and lessened immunity to disease.

Fat in food also combines with oxygen in the bloodstream to form free radicals. Details about free radicals will appear shortly, but for now it's best just to quote Norman Ford's *18 Natural Ways to Look and Feel Half Your Age*: "Along with dietary fat, [free radicals] damage the lining of all arteries and organs within the body and are a major cause of heart disease, stroke, cancer, [and] immunity decline (with a resulting increase in infections)." Jean Carper, in *Stop Aging Now!*, agrees: "This is the stuff aging and disease are made of."

On the other hand, a low-fat diet can defer all of the above conditions.

There are some dissenters. George Washington University's Thomas Moore, in his book *Life Span*, points out that the Swiss, who are the second-longest living people on Earth (after the Japanese), have "more animal fat in [their] diet than virtually any country in the world." Psychologist Robert Ornstein and coauthor David Sobel in the book *The Healing Brain* reported that Japanese immigrants in California had very little heart disease even though their diets varied from low- to high-fat.

Still, Moore says, "lowering the fat . . . is a perfectly sensible idea."

It's impossible to avoid fat entirely. As Stanford's Walter Bortz points out in *Dare to Be 100*, "All foods are fattening."

But as Barnard explains in *Eat Right, Live Longer*, "Some foods go to fat quite easily, while others do not." Bortz says, for example, "One large Snickers bar has as much fat (200 calories) as 50 apples or 120 potatoes."

And even among the fats, some are healthier than others. "Fat is classified according to how saturated or unsaturated it is," says Bortz—saturated, that is, with hydrogen atoms. Among the major fat categories are the following:

SATURATED FAT

The most long-lived people on Earth, the Japanese, have a diet very low in saturated fat. That's a good thing; sat fat can be deadly.

- Barnard says that a woman's risk of ovarian cancer rises by 20 percent with every ten grams of saturated fat in her daily diet. ("That," he says, "is the amount of saturated fat in just 2 ounces of cheddar cheese, 4 ounces of pot roast, or two glasses of whole milk.")

- "Saturated fat," says Ford in *18 Natural Ways*, "promotes the liver to manufacture up to three times its weight in cholesterol. This makes saturated fat the most powerful promoter of cholesterol."

- Says Walford, "Finland, which has the world's highest intake of saturated fats . . . has the world's highest death rate from heart disease."

Saturated fat appears mostly in meat products. Among the meats highest in saturated fat are beef and lamb, says Earl Mindell, Pacific Western University nutrition professor and author of *Earl Mindell's Anti-Aging Bible*. A Burger King Whopper with cheese is 17 percent saturated fat, according to UCLA pathologist Roy Walford, author of the longevity diet book *The Anti-Aging Plan* (written with Lisa Walford).

Dairy can be troublesome, too; the authors of *Live Longer, Live Better* note that Swiss cheese has nine times as much saturated fat as hard-boiled eggs and more than *16* times that of light-meat chicken that's been skinned and broiled.

Oils make the list, too. A hefty *89 percent* of coconut oil is sheer saturated fat, according to the authors of *Age Erasers for Men*. Baked goods, Barnard says, are also rich in sat fat.

And fried foods in general are high in sat fat.

To lower your intake of sat fat, cut down on these foods. When cooking, use low-fat oils. Understand, though, that all oils have some sat fat. For example, canola oil is about as low in saturated fat as any oil you can find, but even it is about 10 percent sat fat.

Entirely avoiding animal products (and their load of sat fat) remains controversial. Several authorities recommend a vegetarian diet to eliminate sat fat, and few dispute that such a diet is a healthy one.

But not every expert *demands* strict vegetarianism. The American Geriatrics Society permits saturated fat watchers to eat fish, skinless chicken, and low-fat dairy products. The authors of *Live Longer, Live Better* say that even red meat is acceptable if you select lean cuts, trim the visible fat, and "roast, bake, or broil the meat on a rack so that the invisible fat drips off." Lovers of dairy foods, says Walford, should try uncreamed cottage cheese, which has very little saturated fat.

But these recommendations are the exceptions. Most experts would side with the Geriatrics Society's *Complete Guide to Aging & Health*, which advises, "Saturated fats should be reduced to less than 10 percent of the total calories [that you consume]."

POLYUNSATURATED FAT

Although most authorities find saturated fat to be the deadliest, Carper disagrees: "The worst fats are polyunsaturated fats and cholesterol."

She goes on, "Studies show polyunsaturated fats foster autoimmune diseases, encourage cancer, help destroy your arteries, and have an adverse affect on your immune function." *Live Longer, Live Better* rates saturated and polyunsaturated fats equally, advising that your consumption of each fat be only 10 percent of your total fat intake.

Carper calls polyunsaturated fat "rancid fat," describing it as an unseen staple in processed foods such as muffins, sauce mixes, pizza crusts, and even vegetable cooking oils. In *Healthy at 100*, heart surgeon Robert Willix says that it's in margarine and mayonnaise. And corn oil ranks among the substances carrying the most polyunsaturated fat: 61 percent of it is polyunsaturated fat, says Carper.

TRANS FATS

When polyunsaturated fats harden, they become trans-fatty acids, also called trans fats—what Carper calls "a kinky new form, unknown in nature."

And deadly. According to Robert Arnot, M.D., in *Dr. Bob Arnot's Guide to Turning Back the Clock*, "Harvard's Dr. Walter Willet believes that these [trans fats] may be two to three times more dangerous than saturated fats."

Trans fats raise cholesterol levels and encourage heart disease. They pack tightly into white blood cells, making the cells so stiff and immobile that they can't attack infections or cancers. Trans fats also clog arteries and promote breast and prostate cancer.

As Willet puts it, "Eating trans fatty acids, particularly margarine, kills from 30,000 to 150,000 Americans every year."

Other foods carrying trans fats are cakes, potato chips, poultry, beef and fried foods. Barnard, in *Eat Right, Live Longer*, points out that trans fatty oils are used in frying foods.

To avoid trans fats, Arnot says, "Avoid products with labels that contain the words *hydrogenated* or *partially hydrogenated*." These words signal that the foods probably contain trans fats.

TRIGLYCERIDES

"If a blood test shows that you have too much fat in the blood, your doctor words this more politely by saying that your triglycerides are elevated," says Barnard. "Triglycerides are special molecules that the body uses to transport fat in the blood and to store it."

Although Barnard notes, "health authorities are not yet sure just how much risk triglycerides pose," *Staying Young* says, "Some scientists believe triglycerides cause the blood to thicken into sludge, reducing blood flow to the heart and other organs." As a result, says Mindell, high triglycerides "are believed to increase the risk of heart attack."

How do triglycerides get into the body? You eat them. As the authors of *Staying Young* note, triglycerides "migrate into the bloodstream when we consume foods rich in fat and sugar." Even fruits have them—although, Barnard notes, triglycerides from fruit and other plants do not increase the risk of heart disease.

Some foods, fortunately, lower triglycerides. Among them are fish oil, capsaicin (a spice also known as cayenne pepper), broccoli, peanuts, mushrooms, brewer's yeast, whole grains (including whole-grain bread), wheat germ, and beans and other legumes.

Dairy foods, eggs, beef, and lamb can also lower triglycerides because they contain such antitriglyceride substances as niacin and L-carnitine. But beware: they can run high in fat.

A logical choice, presumably, would be versions with the lowest possible fat content, such as nonfat milk.

The story of fats sounds ugly. Here's the pretty side.

MONOUNSATURATED FAT

Monounsaturated fat may help to keep you healthy. Mindell says, "In countries such as Italy and Greece, where the diet is rich in monounsaturated fat . . . the incidence of heart disease is a fraction of what it is in the United States." Carper calls monounsaturated fats "the longevity fats."

Although there is some controversy on exactly how effective mono fats are, reputable scientists and journalists contend that they may lower cholesterol levels and stabilize blood sugar levels (thus helping to prevent diabetes).

Olive oil, canola oil, and avocados are strong sources of monounsaturated fats. According to *Age Erasers for Men*, olive oil is the best of the lot; it's a rich 76 percent monounsaturated fat.

"This doesn't mean that you should begin dumping olive or canola oil on your food," says Walford, "since the *total amount* of fats and oils that you eat daily should be kept reasonably low." Even olive oil, for all its mono fat, is 13 to 14 percent saturated fat.

As Mindell warns, monounsaturated fats are still fats: "As beneficial as monounsaturated fats may be, a little goes a long way."

OMEGA-3 FATTY ACIDS

Omega-3 fatty acids are traitors to their class. These fats counteract the destructive power of other fats, the polyunsaturated fats.

Moreover, studies at Dartmouth Medical School reveal that omega-3 acids deter pancreatic cancer. Research at New York Cornell Medical Center shows that omega-3s fight off free radicals.

But the most promising power of omega-3s may be preventing heart and circulatory-system disease.

- University of Washington medicine professor David Siscovick says (according to *Good Housekeeping* magazine), "Eating six ounces of tuna a week is associated with a 50 percent reduced risk of cardiac arrest in men and women."

- Cornell cardiologist Linda Gerber has said, in an article written with anthropologist Douglas Crews of Ohio State University, that omega-3 acids lower cholesterol levels.

- David Ryback's *Look 10 Years Younger, Live 10 Years Longer*—which calls omega-3s "the best of all [fats]"—says, "Omega-3s appear to . . . open the tight pathways of the arteries," adding, "Wider arteries mean less opportunity for heart attacks."

- Walford, noting that omega-3s lessen triglyceride levels, notes that Eskimos have little arteriosclerosis, even though they eat a lot of fat— "but the fat they eat comes mostly from fish." And that fat, says Mindell, "was in the form of omega-3 fatty acids."

Salmon is especially rich in omega-3 acids. Other fish high in omega-3 include sardines, halibut, mackerel, trout, tuna, and herring.

Barnard, who advises that you stay away from fish because it can deliver high amounts of cholesterol, advises eating vegetables rich in omega-3 such as broccoli, spinach, lettuce, and beans. Omega-3 is also available in the herb purslane.

THE BIG PICTURE

For your best antifat eating, avoid:

baked goods	lamb
beef	margarine
coconut oil	mayonnaise
corn oil	poultry (with skin)
fried foods	whole-milk dairy foods

Instead, eat:

avocados	mushrooms
beans	nonfat milk products
brewer's yeast	olive oil
broccoli	peanuts
canola oil	peanuts
capsaicin (cayenne)	skinless chicken
fish and fish oil	spinach
	whole grains

CARBOHYDRATES

Carbohydrates are life extenders. If you want proof, talk to some very old people. "The diet of the longevous contains . . . 70 to 80 percent carbohydrates," says Georgakas.

Carbohydrates keep the body running. Bortz explains, "After a meal, nearly all your energy comes from carbohydrates."

Barnard points out another advantage of carbohydrates: "They cannot add directly to your body fat. There are no little pouches of carbohydrate on your thighs or hips."

COMPLEX CARBOHYDRATES

More than half of the food that you eat in any given day should be complex carbohydrates. "Complex carbohydrates are close to being the perfect food for living ten years longer," says Ryback.

So what is this miracle stuff?

"Complex carbohydrates," says Barnard, "are simply the starchy part of foods: the white insides of a potato, pasta, bread, beans, lentils, and most vegetables."

"Your digestive system breaks down carbohydrates into glucose, [a sugar] which is the body's major source of energy," say the authors of *Live Longer, Live Better*. The body tends to burn complex carbs steadily. Thus, says Arnot, carbs "give you a constant level of mental and physical energy." Since complex carbs are filling, get burned off easily, and are low in fat, "you can actually eat more and still lose pounds," say the authors of the *Age Erasers* books.

Complex carbs are high in fiber. *Age Erasers for Men* mentions that they can fight off diabetes. "Complex carbs also contain potassium," says Barnard, who adds, "people with more potassium in their blood have faster calorie-burning speeds"—that is, they can burn food off of their body before it settles in as fatty deposits.

These carbohydrates can help the mind and emotions as well. Nutritionist Judith Wurtman of the Massachusetts Institute of Technology says that complex carbs can raise levels of the brain chemical serotonin, which can settle moods, calm stress, and erase depression. William O'Connor, M.D., of the State University of New York at Stony Brook notes that complex carbs can help to curb hostility.

Beans and potatoes are thick with complex carbohydrates. Fruits (particularly apples) have complex carbs, as do lentils, air-popped popcorn, peas, sweet potatoes, and cereals. The National Research Council recommends at least five daily servings of fruits and vegetables and six servings of cereal and grain products.

Not all grain products are healthy, though. "Many of them are white-flour products that, to my way of thinking, aren't much better than eating sugar with vitamin pills," Arnot says. "In fact, white bread will raise your blood sugar higher and faster than table sugar and at the same rate as a Mars bar!" Also, says Arnot, "Pastas, grains, breads, and bagels can leave you seriously deficient in muscle-building protein."

Instead, "use whole grains, such as brown rice, as opposed to ground-up grain products, such as pasta or bread," says Barnard. Whole grains such as barley, corn, oats, and rice (especially brown rice) are big sources of complex carbs.

SIMPLE CARBOHYDRATES

Simple carbohydrates, also known as simple sugars, are very good at making the body unhealthy.

The body converts simple carbohydrates into glucose faster than it converts complex carbs. This conversion can give the body a quick blast of energy—the famed "sugar rush"—but the body usually can't use up a big clump of glucose all at once.

Unfortunately, *Live Longer, Live Better* notes, "Excess glucose is stored as fat." Or as Arnot says, eating simple carbohydrates is "like shooting fat into your veins and aiming them at the roll around the middle of your belly."

What's more, Walford points out, simple carbohydrates can speed up glycation, a process in the body that can damage the arteries, nerves, and kidneys.

It's easy to spot the simple carbohydrates. They're in sugars and sugary foods such as candies, cookies, and sodas. "Wholly refined white sugar is the most difficult sugar for the body to handle and should be avoided," says Georgakas. "Partly refined brown sugar, the staple of many health-conscious households, is not much better."

Wherever you find the simple sugars, Georgakas says, "be wary of the various names manufacturers use for sugar." Among those names are:

corn sweetener	maltose
corn syrup	maltodextrin
dextrose	mannitol
fructose	sorbitol
glucose	sorghum syrup
honey	sucrose
lactose	xylitol
levulose	

Are there any relatively safe sugars? Yes. Georgakas says, "The most easily handled and most useful sugars are those found in fruit."

It's best to eat those sugars when they're still inside the fruit. When extracted and added to food (under the name fructose), they may be better than some other sugars—but when you eat them in fruit, you get the many other advantages that come with eating plant foods.

PROTEIN

Most of the body—60 percent of your dry weight, says Bortz—is protein. Muscle, blood, bones, the heart, and the brain are full of protein, and it's part of what helps many cells function. As Bortz puts it, "Protein is who you are."

Proteins are made of the simple compounds called amino acids. Your body can make some of them, but as Bortz says, "there are . . . amino acids that your body cannot make and therefore must be part of your diet." And that's where food comes in.

HOW MUCH PROTEIN DO YOU NEED?

"The minimum daily requirement for adults, established by the Food and Agricultural Organization of the United Nations, are about 30 grams for the average adult female and 38 grams for adult males," says Georgakas. "The National Academy of Sciences in the United States recommends an additional 20 grams as a safety margin."

It's not hard to get that much protein. A balanced varied diet provides all of the protein that you need.

Some foods, of course, have more protein than others.

PROTEIN-RICH FOODS

"The most secure way to obtain . . . essential amino acids is by eating a meat diet," says Bortz. Red meat, poultry, eggs, pork, dairy products, and fish rank high in protein and aminos.

But now comes the catch. Often, these foods have "far more saturated fat than is good for you," says Arnot.

To get protein without a heavy fat load, you can eat the less fatty animal foods. They include egg whites, low-fat yogurt, nonfat cheese, fish (particularly cod, flounder, sole, haddock, halibut, and tuna), shellfish (such as clams, crab, lobster, scallops, and shrimp), and fresh skinless white-meat turkey.

Unfortunately, says Barnard, some of these foods—particularly meats like skinless turkey— "are loaded with what are called sulfur-containing amino acids, which are especially aggressive at causing calcium to be lost." Calcium is crucial to long life.

The body can turn to plants instead—but as Salisbury State University's DiGiovanna writes in *Human Aging: Biological Perspectives*, "Plant proteins often lack or have very little of one or more types [of amino acids]." And as *Live Longer, Live Better* explains, "[Plant] proteins can't be utilized by the body until all [essential] amino acids are present." (The essential amino acids are the ones that the body needs but can't manufacture and must find in food.)

Fortunately, says Bortz, "a vegetarian who is wise and well instructed can totally fulfill the basic amino acid need with a well-conceived collection of vegetables." Not only does *Live Longer, Live Better* report that soybeans contain all of the essential amino acids, but DiGiovanna says "a complete set of amino acids can be obtained from plants by eating specific combinations of plant foods." For instance, according to *Live Longer, Live Better*, "any grain, nut, or seed complements any legume."

Strong sources of plant proteins are rice, legumes (beans and peas, for instance), and grain products such as oatmeal.

WHAT IF YOU GET TOO MUCH?

"Today," says Aronne, "excess protein is a . . . relevant issue for most Americans." In fact, reports *Live Longer, Live Better*, "most Americans consume more than twice as much protein" as they need.

What happens if you get too much protein? "[A] positive energy imbalance may develop," says DiGiovanna.

If that sounds good, it shouldn't. The body has a special form in which it warehouses its unused energy. It's called fat.

(Not everyone necessarily agrees that protein becomes fat. "If you add more protein to your diet, it will likely be eliminated from the body," say the authors of *Staying Young*. That is a minority view, though.)

What's more, excess protein can lead to high blood pressure, coronary artery disease, kidney disease, and cancers of the stomach, breast, prostate, and colon. It can also cause you to lose calcium, a loss that weakens bones.

If you feel that you're getting too much protein, you might cut back on high-protein foods and switch to foods low in protein, such as apples and oils, particularly corn oil and olive oil.

WHEN DO YOU NEED MORE?

You need extra protein if you're getting over a serious disease or injury or undergoing especially hard physical training, says DiGiovanna.

He adds that you need more if your diet is low in amino acids. Signs of such a diet include "structural and muscle weakness, slowed body reactions, increased risk of infection . . . excess bleeding . . . and poor recovery from injury." People with these problems might need more protein—but it's good to check with a doctor before pigging away on steaks.

Do you need more protein in the later decades? That's a controversy. "As you age," notes Bortz, "you need to keep your protein intake high to help offset the loss of muscle tissue." But the American Geriatrics Society disagrees: "It's unlikely that healthy older people suffer significant protein deficiency." When in doubt, check with your doctor.

THE MUSCLE CONTROVERSY

Lean muscle is important to longevity, and protein can build muscle. In fact, says Arnot, "You can't get strong lean high-quality muscle without the right amount of high-quality protein."

True enough. But more protein doesn't necessarily mean more muscle.

The authors of *Staying Young* say: "Contrary to a long-standing myth, nutritionists do not recommend that people increase their protein intake to accommodate a weight-training program. In a normal diet, we get all the protein we need to build strong muscles."

Moreover, says Georgakas, "the actual working of muscle to build new muscle requires energy that is best furnished by carbohydrates and fats."

Thus, for body builders as well as for everyone who wants to live long, the key is not to suck in all the protein that you can. A normal balanced diet will have enough of it.

CHOLESTEROL

Your body needs cholesterol.

That's right. The bogeyman of the bloodstream is essential to proper function.

"Cholesterol," says Barnard, "is the cement that holds cell membranes together." Since the membrane is the skin—or, to continue the cement metaphor, the wall—that holds the cell together, cholesterol is a vital substance. Barnard adds that cholesterol helps the body build hormones and other important secretions.

Cells don't need much cholesterol, though. Bortz notes that your body—primarily, the liver—manufactures 70 percent of the cholesterol that you need. When you eat foods rich in cholesterol (all cholesterol comes from animal foods, by the way), you're giving your body more than it can use.

Excess cholesterol has to go somewhere. Often, it goes into the walls of your arteries. And that's where the trouble begins.

CHOLESTEROL'S POWER

Too much cholesterol can shorten life; less cholesterol can lengthen it.

- A study by the National Heart, Lung, and Blood Institute (the division of the National Institutes of Health that covers heart disease) says that if you lower your cholesterol level, you can lower the chance that you'll die by heart attack.

- "Richard Shekelle, Ph.D., professor of epidemiology at the University of Texas Health Science Center in Houston, found that high-cholesterol eaters . . . cut an average three years off their life spans," says Carper.

- According to a *Journal of the American Medical Association* report, the federal Center for Prevention of Chronic Disease attributed 253,194 deaths to high cholesterol in a single year.

How does this happen? In your arteries, cholesterol builds up masses called plaques. These masses stiffen and thicken the artery walls, making it difficult for blood to flow through the arteries. It's like trying to pass the Johnstown Flood through a garden hose.

Cholesterol can cause atherosclerosis, heart attacks, and lung cancer; it can lower the body's defenses against disease; and it carries poisons such as air pollution throughout your bloodstream.

So cholesterol is to be avoided. Or is it?

THE OTHER SIDE

A minority of authorities claim that cholesterol is not all that fearsome.

In a Finnish study of 1,200 business executives who showed many of the signs of an oncoming heart attack, including high cholesterol, 600 of the men lowered their cholesterol; 600 didn't. But over the next five years, the men with low cholesterol levels died in greater numbers than the ones with high cholesterol.

Moore quotes other sources: the World Health Organization, which found that people taking a cholesterol-lowering drug had an especially high death rate; an article in the *British Medical Journal*, which "showed cholesterol lowering had no effect on total mortality or life expectancy"; and a 1992 editorial in the American Heart Association journal *Circulation*, which said, "We need now to pull back our national policies directed at identifying and treating high blood cholesterol."

Moore feels that cholesterol is not the main culprit in heart disease. Instead, he blames genetics. Chopra believes that emotional stress and exhaustion are the culprits.

Are the dissenters right? No one knows for certain.

For now, though, it may be safer to go with the majority of doctors and cut cholesterol.

HOW TO CUT CHOLESTEROL

Exercise. If you smoke, quit. And avoid stress; as Bortz says, "accountants' cholesterol values go up early in April."

Then there's food. Bortz feels that no one should consume more than 300 milligrams of cholesterol per day. (300 milligrams is the slightest bit more than 1/100th of an ounce.) "With dietary changes alone," reports *Age Erasers for Women*, "you can whittle away an average of 10 percent of your cholesterol reading—and perhaps even more."

How can you get your cholesterol that low? Karen Miller-Kovach, chief nutritionist at Weight Watchers, says "Decreasing saturated fat is the most effective anticholesterol strategy you can use." (Walford notes that the Tarahumara Indians of Mexico and the Yanomamos of Brazil have diets very low in fat—and cholesterol levels under 140, which is a very safe level.)

In particular, Walford and Bortz warn against milk and meat products, and *Age Erasers for Men* blames organ meats in particular. For example, an ounce of beef liver contains (according to Walford) 136 milligrams of cholesterol; a large egg contains 213 milligrams; and a serving of McDonald's scrambled eggs has 399—more than you need in an entire day. Even worse than scrambled eggs, says Walford, are fried or hard-boiled eggs.

Fish is controversial. *Age Erasers for Men* recommends fish for its high level of monounsaturated fat, which can eliminate cholesterol. But Barnard advises staying away from fish altogether: "None are even close to cholesterol-free, and some are extremely high." Given the controversy, it's probably better to keep fish intake moderate.

If you want to eat fish, Barnard lists tuna as one of the better breeds. It has only 10 milligrams of cholesterol per ounce; it's also high in monounsaturated fat. Avoid haddock or rainbow trout, Barnard says, because they have twice as much cholesterol as tuna. Shellfish has even more.

Cut your sugar. "Refined sugars like sucrose (the one in your sugar bowl) tend to increase blood cholesterol," says Walford. *Age Erasers for Women* agrees.

Not all sugars are in your bowl. "If you think you have beaten the cholesterol problem by eating only low-fat foods," says Walford, "you may well be mistaken. Many of those low-fat foods are sweetened, and may for that reason increase internal cholesterol."

On the other hand, plant foods—fruits, vegetables, grains, and even wine, in moderation—are great. "Foods from plants," Barnard says, "are always zero cholesterol."

Some plants can actually lower cholesterol levels. Beans, oat bran, lentils, citrus fruit, peas, apples, barley, walnuts, and garlic can help to do the job.

If diet, exercise, and other methods fail, Willix recommends asking your doctor for anticholesterol treatments.

Know going in, though, that the treatments are not for everyone. Their effect on senior citizens, for example, is not fully known: "All of the studies evaluating cholesterol-lowering drugs have excluded or contained very few older people," reports the American Geriatrics Society's *Complete Guide to Aging & Health*. *Age Erasers for Women* suggests that women take estrogen but warns that it's linked to some cancers.

Even if you do take anticholesterol medications, says Margo Denke, M.D., of the University of Texas's Southwestern Medical Center, don't stop watching your diet. "Drugs aren't a substitute for healthier eating, losing weight, exercising, and other life-style strategies."

GOOD CHOLESTEROL

Another effective way to eliminate cholesterol is to get more of it.

Often, when people refer to cholesterol, they mean LDL—low-density lipoprotein. LDL, says Carper, is the kind that "gets plastered into artery walls."

But there's another kind of cholesterol. HDL—high-density lipoprotein—actually removes cholesterol from tissues, says Walford. It slips the cholesterol into the liver; from there, "it can be either reabsorbed or excreted." As *Age Erasers for Women* puts it, "the HDL carriers are the good guys, rounding up cholesterol and booting it right out of the body."

The result, as cardiologist Willix puts it, is that "HDL protects you from heart disease."

HDL, says Barnard, accounts for about 20 percent of the total cholesterol in most Americans. The experts disagree on exactly how much HDL people should have. The recommendations range from 23 to 33 percent. No matter what number an authority cites, though, virtually everyone favors a high HDL level.

The only exception is for people with very low cholesterol. "If your blood cholesterol is less than 150, you are very unlikely to have a heart attack regardless of the levels of HDL [and] LDL," says Walford.

Most people don't fall into this category and should raise their HDL. "HDL levels can be increased slightly," says Barnard, "by [eating] vitamin C-rich foods." Bortz recommends "a moderate intake of alcohol." And almost all experts recommend exercising and not smoking.

PHYTOCHEMICALS

"The great nutritional discovery of the 1990s," is how Ford describes phytochemicals.

"A newly recognized substance that can add years to your life," Ryback says.

"Key disease-prevention chemicals," Arnot calls them.

In *Aging on Hold*, the *Chicago Tribune*'s Gorner and Kotulak describe them as "a new class of youth-enhancing nutrients that appear to improve gene performance."

So what are they? "Phytochemicals are substances found in plants that may protect them against stresses, climate, and infection, and researchers believe these substances may help people as well," reports *Staying Young*. According to Ford, phytochemicals "protect our bodies against cancer, heart disease, and a host of other degenerative diseases."

There are "several hundred varieties of phytochemicals," says Ford. Two are getting considerable attention at the moment: protease inhibitors and antioxidants.

PROTEASE INHIBITORS

These compounds fight cancer.

Carper says, "A protease inhibitor in soybeans—called the Bowman-Birk inhibitor—is so versatile against various cancers that [Ann Kennedy, Ph.D., of the University of Pennsylvania] calls it 'a universal cancer preventive agent.'"

Protease inhibitors even slow the growths of tumors that have already formed. So promising are protease inhibitors that AIDS researchers are exploring their potential to stop that disease.

Where can you find them? "Protease inhibitors are . . . found not only in soybeans but in most dried beans and all seeds," says Ford.

As important as protease inhibitors are, the phytochemicals that get the most attention are the antioxidants.

ANTIOXIDANTS

Certain foods contain a class of phytochemicals that can shield the body from a pervasive versatile killer. Cardiologist Willix calls that fact "the most important medical discovery of our time . . . as important to the health and well-being of men and women all around the world as was the discovery of penicillin."

During the mid-1950s, the University of Nebraska's Denham Harman, M.D., Ph.D., discovered something evil about one of the most precious substances: oxygen. While the body needs some oxygen to survive, it doesn't need much. "Humans can tolerate breathing pure oxygen for no more than 48 hours," Gorner and Kotulak point out in *Aging on Hold*. "We survive the air we breathe only because it is just 20 percent oxygen." As human bodies age, they can produce too many oxygen molecules—or actually, pieces of them.

Harman discovered that an extra bit of oxygen, known as a free radical, will attach itself to any other molecule. As Michigan State University's Fossel says in *Reversing Human Aging*, the free radical will begin "damaging [the other molecule] by changing its shape and making it useless or dangerous." Free radicals can rust iron, turn foods rancid—and damage human cells.

"When enough [free-radical] damage accumulates," Dr. Earl Stadtman of the National Heart, Lung, and Blood Institute has said, "cells can't survive properly."

Many experts blame free radicals for heart disease, cancer, brain damage, stroke, and other health problems. Carper says, "The free radical theory of aging is so big it encompasses virtually every disease you can think of that comes with increasing age." Free radicals may even cause aging itself; "chances are 99 percent [that free radicals] are the basis for aging," Harman has said.

But not everyone agrees.

The opposition

Initially, the scientific establishment ignored Harman's theory. As he told Kotulak and Gorner, "It sounded like too simple an answer to something as complex as aging." In fact, says Willix, "Dr. Harman's theory was viewed by some to be the product of a crackpot mind. Many gerontologists still aren't convinced that boosting protection against free radicals . . . makes people live healthier longer," say Gorner and Kotulak.

Part of the problem, notes the University of Wales's Bellamy in *Ageing: A Biomedical Perspective*, is that the body can absorb some free radicals and even repair the damage that they cause. Free radicals can even be beneficial. White blood cells can use them to kill bacteria.

But the main obstacle to acceptance of the idea of free radicals, according to health journalist Moore, is that "the free radical theory [is] hard to confirm." As Bellamy explains, "With most diseases, there are no experimental tests to confirm a fundamental role for free radical damage." Bortz notes, "Numerous effects to extend the life span of experimental animals by the use of free radical scavengers [substances that attack free radicals] haven't worked."

Even some of those who find free radicals dangerous doubt Harman's claim that free radicals alone cause aging. Chopra points out, "It has not been shown that older people necessarily have higher levels of free radicals. . . . Free radical damage is but one type of [age-causing] imbalance." A report by ecologist Stephen Weeks (of the University of Georgia) and anthropologists Gillian Bentley (of Northwestern University), Kenneth Weiss, and James Wood (both of Pennsylvania State University), says, "The data do not provide strong support for the claim that [free radical damage] is *the* cause of aging."

Even if free radicals aren't the only cause of aging, many doctors do consider them a risk to health, and foods can fight them.

Stopping the free radicals

Harman and others have fed lab animals antioxidants, substances that the University of California's Hayflick defines in *How and Why We Age* as "chemical inhibitors [that] prevent oxygen from combining with susceptible molecules to form damaging free radicals." The result was that the animals enjoyed a lower rate of premature death than animals without antioxidants.

"Although there is no conclusive evidence that antioxidants are beneficial," says *Live Longer, Live Better*, "studies suggest that they may protect against the diseases of aging."

"Much of your antioxidant protection can come from the foods you already love to eat," says *Age Erasers for Women*. These foods include fruits, vegetables, and grains, especially legumes, leafy green vegetables, and yellow-orange vegetables.

Among the specific foods that experts recommend often are cantaloupe, carrots, spinach, sweet potatoes, and especially (almost unanimously) broccoli. For seasoning, garlic and red peppers get the most recommendations.

But don't fry, says Barnard. And keep away from vegetable oil, red meat, poultry, fish (and fish oils), the dried eggs put in many processed foods, corn oil, safflower oil, margarine, and wine, particularly red wine. These foods promote free radicals.

Though an antioxidant diet can help, Barnard warns, "Foods will not avert or reverse every problem." Other chapters will detail other ways to protect yourself.

But antioxidants are beneficial, and one of the most useful is glutathione.

GLUTATHIONE

"All-important glutathione," is what Carper calls this substance. Memorial Sloan Kettering Cancer Center's John T. Pinto calls it "the master antioxidant." "Glutathione is one of the most important antioxidants produced in the body," agrees Mindell.

Glutathione, it is thought, can help fight cancer, high blood pressure, heart disease, diabetes, infections, and the dangers in alcohol and cigarette smoke.

How does it work? Barnard calls it "the carrier molecule that hauls toxins out of your body." As a result, you live longer.

Sadly, "your blood levels of glutathione drop about 17 percent between ages 40 and 60," says Carper.

How much do you need?

"There is no RDA [recommended daily allowance] for glutathione," says Mindell. But Carper advises 25 to 50 milligrams a day.

It's not hard to get that much. An orange has 10.6 milligrams, a cantaloupe has 9.4, and an avocado a startling 31.3. Other foods with high levels of glutathione include grapefruit, peaches, strawberries, watermelon, cabbage, carrots, and tomatoes.

On the other hand, says Carper, "eating fat boosts your need for glutathione."

So if you eat your fruits and vegetables and avoid fat, you could be lengthening your life in ways that you didn't even know existed.

FIBER

"One thing that advocates for alternative medicine and mainstream groups like the American Medical Association can agree on: Americans should eat more fiber," says Earl Mindell in his *Anti-Aging Bible*. Health journalist Norman Ford says, simply, that fiber "helps us stay young."

Fiber is simply the parts of plants that the body can't digest. Unlike, say, animal fat, it doesn't stay in your body as flab or cholesterol. It speeds through the body and exits as feces, "carrying the bad stuff—like cholesterol, bile acids, and other toxins—out of our system," report the *Age Erasers* books.

Fiber is known to fight cancers of the breast, colon, and bowel. It can fight free radical damage. It can ward off arteriosclerosis, diabetes, constipation, high blood pressure, diverticulitis, obesity, gallstones, and possibly arthritis, hemorrhoids, kidney stones, and stroke. Barnard points out that fiber washes possibly harmful excess hormones out of your body. And it lowers cholesterol levels.

Unfortunately, says Mindell, "The American diet is woefully low in fiber." While most authorities recommend 25 to 40 grams (slightly more than an ounce) of fiber per day, an average American consumes only 10 to 12 grams.

On the other hand, the Chinese average three to four times that amount. They tend to have a cholesterol rate a third lower than the American average, two thirds fewer breast cancers, one fifth as many colon cancers, and less than 10 percent as many heart attacks.

WHERE TO GET IT

"Fiber comes only from plants," says Barnard. "It's what used to be called natural plant roughage." Meats and dairy products, he adds, have no fiber at all.

Vegetables and fruits are good sources of fiber. Among the best are apples, oranges, carrots, beans, broccoli, lentils, peas, and spinach.

Products made from grains can be good, too, particularly oatmeal, wheat bran, oat bran, brown rice, whole wheat bread, and breakfast cereals such as Bran Buds, All-Bran, and Fiber One. The *Age Erasers* books point out that a half cup of All-Bran with Extra Fiber contains 15 grams of fiber, nearly half of what most people need in an entire day and as high an amount as you're likely to find in a half cup of almost anything.

A FEW CAUTIONS

"High fiber alone won't do," the *Age Erasers* books warn. Although fiber can cart some dangerous substances out of your body, don't assume that it allows you to put more bad food in. Fiber just isn't that effective. Fortunately, fibrous foods are pretty filling, so they can cut down your appetite for harmful foods.

"Read labels carefully," say the *Age Erasers* books. "Don't assume that a product with the words 'fiber,' 'bran,' or 'oats' in its title necessarily has the fiber content you're looking for." Look for the phrases "good source of fiber" (2.5 to 4.9 grams of fiber per serving) or "high-fiber" (at least 5 grams)—phrases that the Food and Drug Administration has approved and defined.

"Ease your way gradually into a high-fiber diet," Ford says. Although fiber has no calories and Bortz calls it "cheap and safe," Mindell warns, "If you gobble up too much fiber too quickly, you may develop gas and cramps."

Moreover, says DiGiovanna, too much fiber "can lead to deficiencies in calcium, zinc, and iron, because fiber inhibits the absorption of these nutrients." (As we'll see later, these nutrients can be crucial to long life.)

To relieve such problems, many authorities recommend drinking at least six to eight glasses of water per day, which can wash the fiber out of the body before it can do harm.

Getting fiber in food is better than getting it in supplements. The supplements provide fiber through psyllium ("a purified seed fiber product," says Bortz), the best-known one being Metamucil.

While some experts do recommend supplements, *Age Erasers for Women* says, "they're expensive, and it takes several pills and drinks to equal the fiber content of a piece of fruit." And most experts agree. As Stanford University's Fries says in *Living Well*, "The natural fiber approach . . . is greatly to be preferred over the use of laxatives and bowel stimulants."

FOOD ADDITIVES

"How successfully the body can handle [food] additives is a matter of bitter dispute," says Georgakas. He's right.

On the pro-additive side are the Food and Drug Administration and the Committee on Diet and Health of the National Research Council. They find additives to be safe and even useful.

But an anti-additive view comes from Willix: "Preservatives in food cause free radical damage."

Why do the experts disagree? Says Georgakas, "Different body chemistries have different tolerances for a poison, so there can be no fool-proof safety threshold [of acceptable amounts of additives in food]."

Besides, as Georgakas notes, fruits and vegetables alone can carry "more than 5,000 approved pesticides, waxes, and colorings. With that many additives available, it's easy to find harmless ones and then to turn around and find ones that aren't so harmless. "Potentially dangerous interactions among additives are another concern," says *Live Longer, Live Better*. As Georgakas explains, "chemicals interact when combined, so that taking in several different additives, even those considered safe when taken in isolation, can have unpredictable and possibly adverse chemical consequences."

Moreover, Georgakas notes, the Food and Drug Administration "has been understaffed and underfunded for years," so it cannot monitor every new substance on the market.

Even when the FDA is vigilant, it can't predict unexpected consequences. "No fewer than 14 of the 16 food dyes approved in 1946 were banned in 1980 on the grounds that they were carcinogens," says Georgakas. As *Live Longer, Live Better* notes, "Additives shown to be safe in animal studies may still prove to be harmful over the long term in human use."

For longevity's sake, it's probably best to err on caution's side and stay away from additives whenever possible.

How? Buy food raised without additives. Many stores sell these foods and are proud enough of their wares to label them as such.

Certain additives crop up more often than others. The next several sections explain them.

SWEETENERS

"The most commonly used additives are the sweeteners," says Bortz. They appear in an enormous range of foods, go by many names, and present several life-threatening dangers.

Sugar

As the section on carbohydrates notes, sugar can be hazardous to health. Unfortunately, says Walford, "Sugar is the number one preservative used in today's processed foods." Avoid it when you can.

Artificial sweeteners

These substances are very common—as Bortz says, "The diet drink industry is dependent on aspartame (NutraSweet and Equal) and saccharine"—but how dangerous are they?

Artificially sweetened foods "are not necessarily nutritionally good foods," says Willix. He explains, "artificial sweeteners . . . alter the body's ability to metabolize fat."

Bortz, though, feels that while artificial sweeteners aren't good for you, their dangers may have been exaggerated. "A study showed that bladder cancer occurred in rats when they were fed the equivalent of 850 cans of soft drinks per day, but overall the safety record seems very high."

Individual sweeteners have their own controversies. Aspartame, for example, may alter brain function and behavior, according to *Age Erasers for Women*. Saccharin may encourage cancer and, says Georgakas, "may increase the desire to eat in overweight people . . . [and] intensifies the harmful effects of tobacco."

Given the controversy over these additives, the safe thing to do is to avoid them whenever possible. But what if you still want sweets—and who doesn't?

Safer sweeteners

No sweetener, natural or artificial, seems completely safe. Still, Willix says, "If you need to sweeten your food, use Suc-a-Nat (granulated sugar cane), raw sugar, or natural honey."

Even better, say most authorities, is whole fruit. It's not as much fun as a glazed doughnut, but it can help to stretch your life.

CONTAMINANTS

Two of the best-known and most common life-shortening contaminants are bacteria and pollutants.

Bacteria

"The most dangerous food additive is bacteria that inadvertently contaminates food during storage or preparation," says Bortz. Bacteria cause ailments from diarrhea to death. If food is spoiled or packed in water that's less than clean, then it may breed bacteria.

To avoid bacteria, Bortz advises, "Don't buy foods in damaged wrappers. Eat hot foods hot. Eat cold foods cold. Eat all foods in as fresh a form as possible. Don't overbuy. Watch for expiration dates." *Live Longer, Live Better* adds, "Refrigerate leftovers and other perishables promptly to prevent bacteria from multiplying."

In other words, simply use good sense, and you'll cut your risk of eating dangerous little creatures.

Pollutants

Industrial pollution gets into the air, water, and land. And into the animals and plants that live there. In particular, Georgakas says, "Meat products can have high retention [of pollutants]."

To avoid this problem, *Live Longer, Live Better* recommends, "Avoid organ meats, which contain the highest concentration of toxins. Remove any visible fat before cooking, since toxins accumulate in fat."

Animals that live on land aren't the only source of trouble. "The streams, rivers, and coastal areas where sewage and pesticide runoff end up are exactly where fish live," says Barnard. "According to a 1992 *Consumer Reports* survey, half of the flounder sampled in New York contained pesticides."

"To buy fish, find a reputable fish market that will tell you its fish sources," says *Live Longer, Live Better*. "Buy fish that is displayed unwrapped on ice.... Alternate between deep-water ocean fish, freshwater varieties, and farm-bred fish to limit contamination from a single source. Buy younger, smaller fish, which will have accumulated fewer toxins."

Avoiding contaminants altogether

Go vegetarian whenever possible. As Georgakas says, "The least chemical contamination occurs at the lower end of the food chain. Thus, root vegetables and grains have only a fractional retention of pollutants. . . . Legumes, fruits, and vegetables of all kinds have relatively low retention."

SALT

"For the prolongevous," says Georgakas, "salt, like sugar, should rarely be added to food." The section on sodium—salt is 40 percent sodium—explains why and what to do about it.

SODIUM NITRITE

Sodium nitrite prevents botulism from getting into meat. "Most processed meats contain sodium nitrite and sodium nitrate [a similar substance] as both a preservative and color and flavor enhancer," says Ryback. (In a sense, sodium nitrate might as well be sodium nitrite; *Live Longer, Live Better* notes that cooking and/or digestion turn nitrate into nitrite.)

So far, so good—except that sodium nitrite combines with compounds in the body to become carcinogenic. "Several nations have banned its use," says Georgakas.

"The U.S. Department of Agriculture, which regulates meat and poultry, has banned nitrate from most processed meats and reduced the level of nitrite permitted," says *Live Longer, Live Better*. "But it is still there," adds Ryback.

The solution, the experts agree, is to avoid hot dogs, bacon, and other processed meats whenever possible.

VITAMINS

Vitamins can help to slow the aging process. As Carper says in *Stop Aging Now!*, "Growing old itself—and the diseases that tag along—may be to a large extent a vitamin deficiency disease of incredible magnitude."

Vitamins, says *Age Erasers for Women*, "are organic chemical compounds that act as catalysts." As *Age Erasers for Men* explains, "[Vitamins] facilitate and regulate every biochemical reaction and physiological process."

Vitamins can aid the body in fighting off disease and aging "by boosting antioxidant activity, helping crush the free radicals that are a prime cause of aging," Carper says.

Unfortunately, Ford reports, "Studies by the USDA and other organizations show that older people who eat the standard American diet are often deficient in vitamins A, B_6, B_{12}, folic acid [a B vitamin], C, D, and E." Whatever your age, Carper notes, "You are probably deficient even in the minimal RDA [government-recommended daily adult] requirements for vitamins and minerals. Nearly all Americans are. Thus, you are flirting dangerously with premature aging."

By eating foods that are rich in vitamins, you can slow this process.

A couple of notes before jumping into the facts on various vitamins: "Numerous vitamins and minerals work together to protect against aging," says Carper. "There is no one antiaging miracle vitamin."

Vitamins are available in supplements as well as in foods. Supplements are important but controversial, and another chapter is devoted to them.

VITAMIN A AND THE CAROTENOIDS

"Half of all Americans past 60 are deficient (in vitamin A), even by minimum standards," says Carper.

Vitamin A fights cancer and free radicals. What's more, adds Ryback, "Vitamin A purifies the blood . . . from such pollutants as pesticides, industrial poisons, and the toxic side effects of prescribed medications."

Good sources of vitamin A include milk, liver, eggs, apricots, and watermelon; yellow-orange fruits and vegetables such as cantaloupe, papaya ("each provides almost a complete daily dose of vitamin A," says *Dr. Bob Arnot's Guide to Turning Back the Clock*), carrots, and sweet potatoes; and green leafy vegetables such as spinach, broccoli, collard greens, brussels sprouts, kale, and lettuce.

A warning

Large doses of vitamin A can be dangerous. "Avoid vitamin A," says Barnard. "It can be toxic in even modest overdose and should be avoided unless prescribed by a physician."

The elderly should take special care. The University of Arizona's William Stini says, "A high vitamin A intake can be potentially toxic to the elderly." The American Geriatrics Society's *Complete Guide to Aging and Health* warns, "Too much vitamin A can produce fatigue and weakness, cause liver dysfunction [and] headache . . . and reduce the number of circulating white blood cells."

Large doses of vitamin A usually appear in supplements, not foods. Jeffrey Blumberg, Ph.D., of the U.S. Department of Agriculture's Human Nutrition Research Center says, "We get all the vitamin A we need from meats and vegetables."

In addition to carrots and kale, another safe source of vitamin A is beta carotene.

Beta carotene

Imagine a family of about six hundred. They're all good, but one is exceptional.

The carotene, or carotenoid, family, says Mindell, is a group of compounds that naturally occur in many vegetables. Unfortunately, says Carper, half of all Americans aged 60 and up don't have enough beta carotene, the star of the family and a relative of vitamin A.

Live Longer, Live Better says that the body converts beta carotene into vitamin A— "all the vitamin A the body needs," says Barnard.

Beta carotene boosts immunity, is a stronger antioxidant than vitamin A, and can prevent heart attacks and strokes, fight cholesterol and cancer, and help to keep blood pressure low (although its exact effectiveness at doing these jobs remains in dispute). Walford adds that while vitamin A can be dangerous in large doses, beta carotene is almost completely nontoxic.

How much beta carotene should you consume? At least 5 to 7 milligrams per day, according to the National Cancer Institute.

It doesn't take much to get that amount. Carper notes that a cup of carrot juice has 24.2 milligrams of beta carotene and a medium sweet potato has 10. Beta carotene is common in broccoli, apricot, spinach, pumpkin, cantaloupe, carrots, and, in general, orange-yellow fruits and vegetables and dark-green leafy vegetables.

One last word on beta carotene, this time from Barnard: "If you eat an enormous amount of [beta carotene], it would color you . . . particularly your arms and soles . . . [with] a slight (and harmless) orange tinge."

Other carotenoids

Alpha carotene, lycopene, lutein, zeaxanthin, flavonoids, phenolic acids—these and hundreds of other members of the beta carotene family are effective antioxidants. They're also reputed to fight coronary artery disease and cancer.

Fortunately, they're found in the same foods as beta carotene. So when you eat an orange or some spinach, you're getting a huge variety of life-prolonging natural chemicals.

THE B VITAMINS

Vitamin B is actually several vitamins that are part of what nutritionists call the "B complex": B_1 (thiamine), B_2 (riboflavin), B_3 (niacin), B_6 (pyroxidine), B_{12} (cobalamin), folic acid, and biotin.

"[B vitamins] can alleviate worry over your two most serious concerns as you grow old—your heart and your mental faculties," says Carper. She quotes a study in which "67 percent of the cases of high homocysteine—an artery and brain toxin—among 1,600 elderly men and women was tied to low blood levels of one or more B vitamins." Carper adds that B vitamins can also guard against cancer.

Unfortunately, Ford notes, "The standard American diet remains deficient [in vitamin B]."

Here are the details on what the B vitamins can do and which foods carry them.

Vitamin B_1

"Thiamine, known as B_1, breaks down and converts carbohydrates into glucose, which provides energy for the body," says Mindell. "Thiamine is necessary for the normal functioning of the nervous system, heart, and other muscles."

Elderly people may need more thiamine than the young, writes the University of Arizona's William Stini in the collection *Biological Anthropology*. He cites an Irish study in which old women who went from low to high thiamine levels had a better appetite, higher energy, and, overall, more activity. Activity, as another section of this book details, is often crucial to a long life.

Thiamine is common in whole-grain products, especially cereals. It's also in pork, brewer's yeast, nuts, and legumes such as beans and green peas.

Be careful in cooking thiamine-rich foods. They won't hurt you—Mindell says, "Thiamine has no known toxic effects"—but, he notes, "Thiamine is easily destroyed by exposure to light and heat." Lastly, he says, "Thiamine can be destroyed by alcohol."

Vitamin B_2

Like B_1, vitamin B_2 (also known as riboflavin), helps the body digest foods and release energy to the body's cells. "Riboflavin may also protect against certain forms of cancer and oxidative damage by free radicals," says Mindell.

Dairy foods, leafy vegetables, and enriched grains are strong in B_2.

Vitamin B₃

B$_3$ helps the digestive and nervous systems, and the body's cells need it to use oxygen. Mindell notes that it may help to prevent heart attacks and cancer.

In high amounts, says Ryback, niacin reduces overall cholesterol levels, including that of LDL (the "bad" cholesterol), while raising the level of HDL ("good" cholesterol).

In high amounts, niacin can, unfortunately, encourage diabetes in elderly people, reports *Staying Young*—but high amounts come primarily from supplements. As *Staying Young* says, "There's no danger from niacin in your diet. You can't get enough of it from food to cause a [diabetic] reaction."

But niacin can drive health-conscious people nuts. For example, milk and eggs are high in niacin—but they're also high in fat and cholesterol. Mindell notes, "As people cut back on high-fat and high-cholesterol foods, such as milk and egg products, they may become deficient in niacin." What's an eater to do?

Fortunately, enriched-grain and whole-grain breads are rich in niacin. If they don't help, ask your doctor about supplements.

Vitamin B₆

This vitamin can help the body prevent cancer. It strengthens the immune system's fight against infection. It contributes to keeping the heart healthy and the blood supply fresh. And it helps to prevent the declining mental state that sometimes comes with age.

"You can get the RDA [government recommended daily allowance] of 1.6 milligrams of B$_6$ by eating two large bananas," report the *Age Erasers* books. B$_6$, otherwise known as pyridoxine, also crops up in fish, prunes, whole grains, poultry, walnuts, and sweet potatoes.

Vitamin B₁₂

B$_{12}$ helps the body produce red blood cells, keeps the nervous system functioning, prevents lung cancer, and metabolizes protein and fat. But its most important power may be to keep the brain functioning.

Mindell notes, "B_{12} has been touted as the 'brain vitamin' because a lack of this important vitamin can severely hamper mental agility." Specifically, confusion and dementia can arise from low levels of B_{12}.

Animals produce B_{12}, and dairy products, poultry, and fish are good sources of the vitamin. Plants, generally, are not.

Fortunately for vegetarians, "the recommended dietary allowance [of B_{12}] is minuscule—only 2 micrograms per day," says Barnard. Two micrograms amount to less than a ten-millionth of an ounce. "Breakfast cereals and other packaged foods are sometimes enriched with B_{12}, which may be listed among the ingredients by its chemical name, cobalamin or cyanocobalamin."

Elderly people may not be able to absorb B_{12} no matter how much they eat. Atrophic gastritis, a condition common in the elderly, lessens the amount of stomach acids that help the body to absorb B_{12} from food. Fortunately, B_{12} supplements can help people who suffer from atrophic gastritis.

Folic acid

"If your cells run low in folic acid, you can kiss your youth goodbye," says Carper. Mindell agrees: "It's for people of all ages, especially those who want to live to be a ripe old age."

Although it's not named B-something, folic acid (also known as folate or folacin) is a B vitamin. It may help to prevent heart disease, cancers of the colon and cervix, memory loss, depression, and dementia. It helps the body make red blood cells, repair tissues, and maintain immunity to disease.

And now, the bad news. "Western diets are often low in folate," says Barnard. "Women on average get only one-half of the recommended daily allowance" of folic acid—the RDA being 400 micrograms.

To get your folic acid (and doesn't that sound like a cheery prescription!), consume leafy green vegetables such as spinach; legumes such as beans, especially dried beans; and citrus fruits, particularly oranges and/or orange juice.

Something that you shouldn't ingest—at least, not much—is alcohol. "Alcohol and other drugs can interfere with the body's absorption of folic acid," reports the American Geriatrics Society's *Complete Guide*.

Biotin

Biotin helps the body absorb the fats, proteins, and carbohydrates in foods. Although not as crucial to longevity as B_{12} or B_6, it does help the body work. Good sources of biotin include poultry (including eggs) and vegetables such as cauliflower and lentils.

VITAMIN C

Vitamin C is an antioxidant.

It can help your body produce glutathione and absorb vitamin E (another antioxidant).

It can help you prevent cancer and heart disease.

It raises HDL ("good") cholesterol levels and lowers LDL ("bad") cholesterol.

Lowering blood pressure, empowering the immune system, strengthening muscles, healing wounds and broken bones, preventing diabetes, and improving lung function—vitamin C helps the body do all of these things.

"One-fourth of all Americans do not get even the minimal, rock-bottom amount of 60 milligrams of vitamin C that cells need," says Carper. Fortunately, several foods are rich in the stuff. "One 8-ounce glass of fresh orange juice may provide up to 100 milligrams of vitamin C," Ford says. Other C-rich foods are strawberries, cantaloupe, brussels sprouts, broccoli, cauliflower, kiwi fruit, sweet potato, peppers, and citrus fruits, particularly oranges.

VITAMIN D

Vitamin D can help to prevent stroke as well as cancers of the colon, rectum, breast, and prostate. But its most renowned function involves bones.

A lack of vitamin D can lead to osteoporosis, a rapid loss of bone matter, which shrinks bones and makes them easily breakable—and which, Mindell says, "can be very serious, even fatal." Even if osteoporosis doesn't kill, it makes exercise difficult; and as later chapters will show, exercise is important to living a long life.

Sunlight, to be discussed in a later chapter, is a good source of vitamin D. "Only if we are deprived of sunlight do we need to worry about sufficient levels of this [vitamin]," says Ryback.

But not everyone can get the right amount of sunlight (from 15 to 105 minutes per week, depending on factors such as age, sex, and location). In that case, "be sure you're getting enough vitamin D from dietary sources," suggest the *Age Erasers* books.

Among the foods rich in vitamin D are eggs, fish (particularly salmon, sardines, and tuna), and vitamin D fortified milk.

Two warnings: Some people don't absorb vitamin D well from milk. Also, large amounts of vitamin D can be poisonous, although those amounts appear in supplements rather than food.

VITAMIN E

This vitamin is a powerful antioxidant, especially when working in combination with vitamin C and beta carotene.

Vitamin E can help the body protect itself against cancer, stroke, heart attacks, and hardened arteries. It may help to protect the body against diabetes, senility, infections, viruses, and air pollution and other airborne poisons.

What can't vitamin E do? Unfortunately, as *Search for Immortality* notes, "its efficacy as a sex vitamin has been disproved."

Good sources of vitamin E include beans, nuts, leafy green vegetables (particularly broccoli, brussels sprouts, and kale), plant oils (especially sunflower oil), sweet potatoes, wheat germ, and whole grains.

VITAMIN K

Perhaps the least-known vitamin, K "is attracting the attention of researchers worldwide because of the possible role it may play in helping to prevent osteoporosis," says Mindell. Vitamin K may help bones retain calcium, the major building block of bones.

Moreover, since it helps the blood to clot, "deficiency of vitamin K is a common cause of bleeding problems in older people," reports the American Geriatrics Society's *Complete Guide to Aging and Health*. And, says *Live Longer, Live Better*, vitamin K "may help to prevent some cancers."

Good sources of vitamin K are eggs and green leafy vegetables such as broccoli and cabbage.

MINERALS

What are minerals for? Salisbury State University's DiGiovanna puts it simply and elegantly: "Minerals are needed so that the body cells can perform properly."

For details on various minerals and the foods in which they appear, read on.

BORON

This mineral has two uses.

"Boron . . . helps keep calcium in the bones," says Barnard. "Researchers at the U.S. Department of Agriculture found that [boron] could double serum estrogen levels in women, which could help to prevent osteoporosis," says Mindell. "In both sexes, boron appears to help the body maintain the essential minerals necessary to prevent bone loss."

Boron also helps the mind.

- Mindell mentions an Agriculture Department study in which men and women on a low-boron diet "displayed impaired mental functioning when asked to perform simple tasks such as counting and tapping."

- *Staying Young* claims that boron helps memory. "Several studies have shown that low dietary and blood levels of iron, zinc, and boron can compromise memory function."

- The *Age Erasers* books list a study in which people "who ate high-boron diets . . . scored higher on tests of attention and memory."

All of the experts agree that the body doesn't need much boron; for example, the *Age Erasers* books note that the full daily amount is contained in three apples. Other sources include vegetables (especially legumes), nuts (especially peanuts), and dried fruit (especially prunes).

CALCIUM

Calcium's main power is strengthening bones. "Calcium is to your bones what air is to your lungs—the element they need to be healthy," says *Age Erasers for Women*. "About 90 percent of the minerals in the matrix [the bony part of bone matter rather than the marrow or blood vessels] consist of calcium and phosphorus," says DiGiovanna.

Calcium has other jobs, too. It helps to keep blood pressure normal, to protect against cancer and strokes, to keep cells working properly, to make nerves and muscles function, and it may even fight LDL ("bad") cholesterol.

But there's a catch. Stini, who calls bones "the ultimate reservoir of calcium," notes, "The physiological functions of calcium are assigned a higher priority than its structural role as a component of . . . bone mineral." *Age Erasers for Women* puts it more clearly. "When your body calls on its daily dose of calcium and can't find it in food, it plucks it from your bones."

As a result, "a relative deficiency of calcium has . . . been suggested as a cause of [the bone-weakening disease] osteoporosis," says the American Geriatrics Society's guide. "About 650,000 fractures occur each year in the United States as a result of osteoporosis," Fries reports in *Living Well*.

A U.S. Department of Agriculture survey has declared that most

Americans don't get enough calcium. According to various estimates, 10 to 50 percent of all Americans lack the calcium that they need.

Fortunately, getting more calcium isn't difficult. "Food is the best way to get calcium," says *Age Erasers for Women*. Fries advises four servings a day of calcium-rich foods.

Good sources of calcium include milk; fish such as salmon and sardines (with bones); figs; tofu; calcium-fortified orange juice; mustard greens; turnip greens; collard greens; nuts (especially almonds); dark-green leafy vegetables such as broccoli, brussels sprouts, bok choy, and kale; various beans (such as pinto beans, white beans, and soybeans); cheeses; and grains.

How much of these foods do you need? With that question, the arguments begin. Recommendations range from the World Health Organization's 400 to 500 milligrams per day to the National Osteoporosis Foundation's 1,000 to 1,600 milligrams.

"One of the reasons that the [proper daily amount] of calcium is difficult to determine," says *Live Longer, Live Better*, "is that [age] can affect its absorption. . . . Children absorb up to 75 percent of the calcium they eat; adults, only 15 to 35 percent." So the older you are, the more calcium you need.

Another problem is that even if you take in a lot of calcium, you may also need to eliminate the substances that block your bones from absorbing it. These substances are so powerful that, as Stini puts it, "Calcium absorption rises very little with increasing calcium intake." Or as Walford puts it in discussing the Chinese, "Their diet includes only half as much calcium as ours (they eat hardly any dairy products), yet they are at a much lower risk for osteoporosis."

Take meat, for example. It's acidic; to neutralize the acids in meat protein, the body sucks calcium from the bones. Or as Barnard puts it, "If you want to weaken your bones, have a chicken salad sandwich."

Sodas, coffees, teas, and other drinks with caffeine are enemies of calcium. Phosphorus—contained in soft drinks, eggs, and meat—also hinders calcium absorption, as does fat in foods. Edibles rich in sodium, such as any salty foods, also reduce calcium. Even spinach, a food high in calcium, contains compounds called oxalates that can reduce the body's ability to absorb the mineral.

But all is not lost. If you avoid salt, fat, caffeine, and meat—good things to avoid or reduce in any case—and turn to most green vegetables, your bones should have all the calcium they need.

CHROMIUM

Chromium aids the body in regulating blood-sugar levels and in burning fat. It may help the body prevent heart disease and diabetes, and strengthen the immune system.

Most importantly, chromium can prevent you from having too much of the hormone insulin in your blood, says Carper. Insulin can destroy arteries, raise levels of "bad" cholesterol, and push the body toward diabetes and maybe even cancer.

Some troubling news: "Chromium is more likely to be in short supply in the American diet than any other substance," says Ryback. And, Mindell says, "As we age, we need this mineral more than ever."

Good food sources of chromium include brewer's yeast, mushrooms, peanuts, broccoli, and whole grains, particularly whole wheat.

Even if you eat those foods, you may not get enough chromium because sugar depletes the chromium in your body and makes it less powerful. To retain your chromium, go light on sugar.

A version of chromium called chromium picolinate has made rats in laboratory tests live much longer than rats ordinarily do. Whether or not chromium picolinate can have so powerful an effect in humans remains to be seen—but the ability of chromium to ward off diabetes and heart disease is powerful in itself.

IRON

"Excess iron can be very dangerous," Denham Harman, discoverer of free radicals, has said. "Excess iron is a true poison," University of Oklahoma hematologist Sylvia Bottomley advises. "Even a little too much," claims Barnard, "can mean serious problems."

Iron can create free radicals. It helps cholesterol attack cells. It's involved in cancer, atherosclerosis, diabetes, and cirrhosis of the liver. It's especially busy at encouraging heart disease; DiGiovanna notes, "Some scientists think [iron] provides a risk [of heart disease] exceeded only by smoking."

Not everyone faces these problems. Children, adolescents, and women before menopause (especially pregnant women) need iron.

So do some older people. The American Geriatrics Society's guide explains that a low level of hemoglobin, the component of red blood cells that carries oxygen, can cause anemia. Anemia in turn can cause fatigue, weakness, shortness of breath, dizziness, pallor, apathy, confusion, agitation, and depression. And a cause of anemia is too little iron in the bone marrow, where red blood cells are formed.

Although having too little iron can cause big problems, Carper claims that too much iron can create even bigger ones. (Moreover, notes the American Geriatrics Society, even people with high levels of iron in their diet can have anemia.)

Fortunately, says Carper, "All you need is a low-maintenance dose [of iron] to keep things running smoothly." To keep the body's stores of iron at safe levels, the experts recommend various methods.

Eating plants, for example. The body can handle and discard excess iron from plant sources—known as non-heme iron—more easily than from animal sources. Plants strong in non-heme iron include legumes, especially beans and peas, and dark-green leafy vegetables. (Popeye was right: Spinach is high in iron.)

Carper notes that tea, bran, and beans can prevent the body from absorbing iron. Calcium is effective, too, says Stini: "The calcium in milk and cheese can interfere with iron absorption."

Donating blood, says Barnard, can also lower iron absorption. In a way, that's why young women don't have much trouble with excess iron: they get rid of it via blood loss in menstruation.

Red wine is controversial. Carper says that it can block iron absorption. But Barnard says that red wine "is also loaded with iron . . . [and] causes the body to absorb even more iron." Check with your doctor about red wine.

Finally, when cooking, "avoid uncoated iron cookware," says Barnard. Food can leach iron from pots and pans.

MAGNESIUM

Magnesium can help to keep the heart healthy, prevent diabetes, maintain normal blood pressure and strong bones, fight free radicals, and break up blood clots. It helps the muscles and nerves work. It helps the body change sugar to energy and absorb calcium, vitamin C, and potassium.

"Unfortunately, America's intake of magnesium has been dropping for a century, since we started processing foods and robbing them of their trace elements [such as magnesium]," report the *Age Erasers* books. "Chances are great that you don't get enough magnesium," says Carper. "Only one in four Americans gets the recommended daily allowance. . . . Two-thirds of older people, who need it most, consume less than 75 percent of the RDA for magnesium."

"You could get the current 300-milligram RDA [recommended daily allowance] dose from just a serving of bran cereal and nuts per day," says Carper (although she finds 300 milligrams "far too low"). In addition, dark-green leafy vegetables such as spinach are rich in magnesium, as are legumes (especially lima beans), whole grains, low-fat milk, potatoes, and bananas.

A caveat: "Too much magnesium can give you a nasty case of diarrhea," say the *Age Erasers* books. Supplements are likelier than food to cause this problem.

POTASSIUM

Potassium keeps your heart beating regularly. It speeds up the rate at which you burn calories, thus helping you to lose weight. It helps to keep calcium from being leached out of bones. It aids the muscles, nerves, kidney, and heart in functioning. It may lower the risk of stroke.

But the mineral's most important job is in handling high blood pressure. "In [potassium's] *absence,* blood pressure goes up," Ryback notes.

Elderly people are especially susceptible to low potassium. "Between the second and ninth decades [of life], there is a loss of 60 percent" of the potassium in body fluids, says Bellamy in *Ageing: A Biomedical Perspective.*

Gender is important, too, Bellamy adds: "At all ages, men have significantly greater amounts of body potassium than women."

Be careful with coffeee; it can lower potassium levels, as can diuretics. Diarrhea, vomiting, hypoglycemia (low blood sugar), or gastrointestinal disorders can make potassium levels drop.

The *Age Erasers* books recommend getting 3,500 milligrams of potassium a day. "It's easy to get enough," the books say. "A baked potato packs 838 milligrams of potassium all by itself, and one cup of spinach has 800 milligrams."

Other strong sources of potassium include fruit (particularly bananas and oranges), milk, yogurt, and vegetables such as broccoli and beans.

Although an overdose of potassium is not likely to come from foods and would not usually be fatal in any case, it can cause kidney problems. "People with kidney disease," says Mindell, "should not take a potassium supplement or consume foods high in potassium."

SELENIUM

Selenium can help the body prevent cancer, heart disease, vulnerability to viruses, stroke-inducing blood clots, high cholesterol levels, circulatory disease, and free radical damage.

How does this mineral do all these things? For one thing, it's an antioxidant—but it also helps other longevity substances do their own jobs.

- "Selenium is not only an antioxidant on its own," adds Carper. "It is an essential building block for the creation of glutathione peroxidase, one of the body's most critical enzymes, [which] neutralizes free radicals."

- Mindell adds that selenium increases the antioxidant power of vitamin E, and vice versa.

- And, according to Carper, selenium helps the body synthesize coenzyme Q-10, which "helps correct deficiencies that come with age, particularly related to your heart, brain, immune functioning, and general resistance to chronic diseases."

Other experts are not quite so enthusiastic. Walford, for example, says, "the evidence for [selenium] having a life span prolonging effect is marginal." But even he praises its power to delay the onset of cancer and heart attack.

Some people need more selenium than others. "As you age," Carper warns, "your levels of selenium fall." She adds that if you don't have much selenium in your body, you're more likely to develop heart disease or cancer than people with adequate selenium. "A lack of selenium can turn viruses from benign to very ugly, able to trigger mechanisms that allow them to replicate and cause illnesses."

Fortunately, as Moore puts it in *Life Span*, "Western diets contain more than adequate amounts of selenium." It's in garlic, tuna, whole-grain breads and cereals, and chicken.

Selenium comes from the soil, and the amount found in different regions varies widely. That could be a serious problem, but it needn't be. "You might not get enough selenium if your sources for it were all from the same geographic location," says Barnard. "But if your bread comes from Kansas wheat, your spaghetti from North Dakota, and your biscuits from France, there is an averaging effect . . . and you are almost certain to get plenty of selenium."

But be careful with selenium. "Selenium can be toxic (hair loss, liver damage, joint inflammation) in high doses," says Carper. "Very high doses can impair immune responses," adds *Age Erasers for Women*.

Although these doses generally come in supplements rather than foods, Carper notes, "Even excessively eating Brazil nuts [a generous selenium supplier] could be toxic to the liver."

"A much better strategy," says Barnard, "is to be sure that your diet contains generous amounts of bread, rice, pasta, cereals, and other grains. This will provide enough selenium to protect your cell membranes [from free-radical damage] but will avoid excesses."

SODIUM

This is serious stuff.

"A high blood sodium level is . . . a marker of serious illness and carries a high death rate," says the American Geriatrics Society's guide. Sodium raises blood pressure by stiffening and aging the arteries. Heart and circulatory-system diseases follow.

Finding sodium is easy. "The vast majority of our sodium intake," report the *Age Erasers* books, "is from the salt in our foods (table salt is about 40 percent sodium)."

Some people are more sensitive to salt than others. If you're overweight, don't exercise, have a family history of high blood pressure or diabetes, or are simply old, you're probably sensitive to salt and should cut down on it.

The National Academy of Sciences advises that adults get at least 500 milligrams of sodium per day. One fourth of a teaspoon of salt carries that much sodium; so do fish, dairy products, eggs, and meats.

A maximum intake should be no more than 2,400 to 4,000 milligrams per day, and it's probably safest to stay as low as possible.

Unfortunately, say the *Age Erasers* books, "Most of us are eating about two and a half times more [sodium] than we should."

Fast food—such as chicken nuggets (up to 140 milligrams of sodium apiece), hamburgers (up to 1,800 milligrams), and ham and cheese sandwiches (1,655 milligrams)—is among the highest in sodium content. Other high-sodium foods include pickles, cookies, potato chips, sodas, soy sauce, cheese, soup and broth, bread, salad dressings ("opt for vinegar and oil over other dressings whose contents you can't find out," says *Age Erasers for Women*), and even milk and ice cream.

- "Restrict processed foods," Carper says. "They contribute about 70 percent of sodium to typical diets."

- "When eating in restaurants," advises *Live Longer, Live Better*, "avoid foods that are smoked, barbecued, or marinated."

- At home, says *Staying Young*, cook with liberal quantities of chopped onions, garlic, basil, and oregano instead of salt, and use vinegar, lemon and lime juice, herbs, and spices.

Be careful in reading food labels. *Reduced sodium* or *less sodium*, says Ryback, means "at least 25 percent less sodium per serving than the usual product." If the usual product is high in sodium—say, a small microwave pizza, at 560 milligrams—then a reduced-sodium version could still have a heavy 420 milligrams.

Instead, look for other labels. *Low sodium* means 140 milligrams or less per serving. *Very low sodium* means 35 milligrams or less per serving. And foods marked *sodium free* aren't necessarily sodium free; they can contain up to 4 milligrams of sodium per serving.

Some foods don't need labels. Apples, bananas, oranges, grapefruit, rice, and navy beans all have less than three milligrams of sodium per serving.

Still, Carper warns, "Reducing sodium is not a universal cure-all." If sodium levels drop too far too fast, you could face fatigue, weakness, confusion, nausea, and muscle cramps.

What can cause such a drop in sodium levels? Excessive sweating, vomiting, diarrhea, and drugs, especially diuretics.

Or something worse. "A low sodium level often reflects a serious problem because it occurs in advanced disease states," says the American

Geriatrics Society. "For example, people may develop a low sodium [level] when they have significant heart, liver, or lung disease, or cancer that has spread widely. For people in the hospital, it means a poor outlook and a sevenfold increase in death."

But for most people who want to live a long time, the greater danger is high sodium. And the best solution is simply to eat right.

ZINC

Zinc is another antioxidant. It can fight cancer and brain disease and help the body repair damaged tissues. Dr. Terry Phillips of George Washington University Medical Center says, "Of all the minerals, zinc is probably the most important for maintaining immunity."

Old people tend to get insufficient amounts of zinc. Carper notes, "One in three healthy Americans over age 50 has a zinc deficiency and rarely suspects it." The reason for the deficiency is "probably . . . a combination of reduced intake and reduced absorption [into the body]," says Stini.

Vegetarians should watch their zinc, too. Since zinc is mostly in meat, seafood, and poultry, a vegetarian diet that's not well-planned or well-balanced could lead to a zinc deficiency.

Good sources of zinc are meat, especially poultry and eggs; grains, especially wheat germ; legumes, especially beans; and seafood, especially oysters. (Carper calls oysters "the richest source [of zinc] known"—which may have something to do with those legends of oysters being aids to sexual potency; low zinc levels in men lead to a low sex drive.)

A couple of warnings. "Cereals, nuts, and seeds are relatively high in zinc, but they also contain agents that reduce zinc absorption [in the body]," says Carper. In other words, they give you lots of zinc but keep you from using it.

And an excess of zinc can be toxic, says Barnard. But, he notes, the body is likelier to overdose on zinc from supplements rather than from foods.

HORMONES IN FOOD/
FOOD'S EFFECTS ON HORMONES

Hormones in food can affect your life expectancy—and food can affect the hormones in your body.

Exactly what are hormones? "Hormones," explains the *Random House Encyclopedia*, "exercise chemical control of body functions, regulating virtually all body functions—growth, development, sexual maturity and functioning, metabolism, [and] emotional balance."

As a result, hormones may influence longevity. As Chopra declares, "It is likely that many of the most important age changes are mediated by hormones."

HORMONES IN FOOD

"Sex hormones themselves can find their way into foods," Barnard explains. "If you were to look behind the ear of a steer on just about any American farm, you would find a small implant about the size of the end of a sharp pencil. The implant contains hormones that make cattle grow faster."

He adds: "Dairy products contain sex hormones, too. . . . The hormones circulating in a pregnant cow's blood easily pass into her milk."

The result, Barnard says, is that "several population studies have shown a correlation between dairy product consumption and breast cancer incidence."

The solution is to avoid beef and milk from cows that were raised with bovine growth hormone or other hormones. Instead, patronize food stores that advertise hormone-free meat.

FOOD'S EFFECT ON HORMONES

Some foods promote hormone excesses in the human body even if the foods themselves aren't hormone-injected.

"In the human body, hormones are stored in fatty tissue," says

Mindell. "Therefore, it's possible that a diet high in fat could result in more fat stores in the body and higher levels of hormones."

So, Barnard advises, "Cut the fat. . . . Reducing the amount of fat you eat helps eliminate hormone excesses."

While fat can raise hormones, plants can control them. "A low-fat, vegetarian diet . . . smoothes out the hormone ups and downs," says Barnard. Moreover, the fiber in plants can carry excess hormones out of the body.

"A plant-based diet has another surprising effect," says Barnard. "It increases the amount of sex hormone binding globulin (SHBG) in the blood. SHBG is a protein molecule that . . . holds the estrogen or testosterone . . . until [it is] needed. It keeps sex hormones in check."

The problem with hormones is that some authorities warn against raising your level of hormones, while others warn against letting them fall too low. Besides, there are several different kinds of hormones in the body, and few authorities specify a proper level for each.

The proper level of hormones in your body is a topic to discuss with your doctor. In the meantime, here's a guide to the ways in which hormones affect you, and how food affects hormones.

ESTROGEN

The female hormone estrogen directly affects longevity. As journalist Carol Orlock says in *The End of Aging*, "Estrogen tends to protect women against heart disease and keep their bones strong."

Orlock explains, "Women's risk of heart disease is low in the years before menopause, but once their estrogen levels drop, the risk rapidly rises." As Hayflick notes, "This is the basis for the belief that estrogen may have some protective effect on the cardiovascular system." Among the possibilities are that estrogen seems to lower the level of LDL ("bad") cholesterol and raise the level of HDL ("good") cholesterol.

As for bones, Fossel lays out the process as follows: "Estrogen loss, after menopause, is like taking the brake off bone loss; bone destruction moves into high gear, bone formation has been slowing with age, and the pool of total bone falls imperceptibly, but steadily." (DiGiovanna adds that men don't suffer the same problem because their bones don't depend on estrogen for strength.)

So too little estrogen can mean trouble. Unfortunately, so can too much. High levels of estrogen can cause breast cancer.

Which foods affect estrogen production?

Alcohol is one.

- Women who drink about an ounce of pure alcohol daily (about two average drinks) have higher amounts of estrogen in their blood and urine than when they don't drink, according to *The Journal of the National Cancer Institute.*

- A study of 128 women cited in *Age Erasers for Women* found that those who had three to six drinks a week had levels of natural estrogen that were 10 to 20 percent higher than women who didn't drink.

- "Two mixed drinks per day can increase a woman's estrogen levels by 30 percent," says Barnard.

Water may be troublesome, too. "Chlorine and related chemicals [in drinking water] can mimic the effects of estrogens," says Barnard. "No one knows how much risk there may be, but the U.S. Environmental Protection Agency is concerned enough that it is looking into other methods of water disinfection."

To avoid this problem, Barnard suggests using bottled water for drinking and cooking and reserving tap water for other household needs.

But the most important dietary cause of high estrogen levels is animal fat. Mindell says, "Vegetarian and semivegetarian women have a much lower rate of breast cancer than women who eat meat."

Why is this? It's not just the fault of hormone-injected cows. Some other reasons are:

- Plant fiber, such as is found in wheat bran, may bind with estrogen and take it out of the body with the feces.

- Soybeans, soy products, alfalfa, apples, barley, and legumes (particularly peas), says Barnard, "contain phytochemicals [that] attach to microscopic receptors [for estrogen] on cells, displacing some of a woman's normal estrogen. The result is less estrogen stimulation and apparently less cancer risk."

- Mindell says that cabbage, broccoli, brussels sprouts, kale, and cauliflower have indoles, a group of phytochemicals that can prevent estrogens from causing cancer.

- Red and yellow onions as well as shallots have quercetin, a substance that can slow the growth of estrogen-related tumor cells, Mindell says.

So to control estrogen-related cancer, eat plant foods.

PROGESTERONE

The other major female sex hormone is much like estrogen—but more so. "Progesterone," Barnard says, "does not just slow bone loss; it actually *builds* bone." Moreover, he says, "Progesterone can increase the sex drive in women . . . (and) does not appear to increase cancer risk."

Without progesterone, trouble can develop. According to *Live Longer, Live Better,* the natural reduction in progesterone that follows menopause "can cause such problems as accelerated bone loss [and] increased risk of heart disease and breast cancer."

Some plants offer natural progesterone. Yams are probably the best-known source.

TESTOSTERONE

In the 1890s, notes *Search for Immortality,* Viennese professor Eugen Steinach noticed that testosterone seemed to give men youth and vitality.

So he encouraged men to have vasectomies in order to keep testosterone from leaving their bodies.

Steinach's methods were wrong, but he was right to notice that testosterone can influence longevity.

A lean muscular body is likely to live a long time, and *Aging on Hold* notes that testosterone "is an efficient muscle builder." It can also, says DiGiovanna, help to thicken and strengthen bones.

Less certain is testosterone's role in heart disease.

- "Testosterone," reports *Live Longer, Live Better,* "lowers the level of high-density lipoproteins (HDLs), the 'good' cholesterol that helps protect against heart disease."

- But, Mindell counters, "One important study performed at Saint Luke's-Roosevelt Hospital Center in New York showed that contrary to previous assumptions, men with lower levels of testosterone were more likely to get heart disease than men with higher levels. In addition, men with higher testosterone levels had higher levels of high-density lipoproteins."

The jury remains out on this topic.

Something neither as life-enhancing as building strong muscles or as ambiguous as testosterone's effects on the heart is its power to promote cancer. As Barnard puts it, "Testosterone and related hormones stimulate prostate cancer cells like fertilizer on weeds."

Finally, testosterone can get the whole body killed. *Aging: A Natural History* points out that among animals, "aggressive behavior is often increased by high testosterone." Not that testosterone affects humans in exactly the same way that it affects animals—but excessive aggression, as history shows, has killed many humans.

Among the foods that raise testosterone levels are fast-burning, easily digestible carbohydrates such as sweet potatoes, says Arnot. Moreover, says Mindell, zinc stimulates the production of testosterone. As noted earlier, you can find zinc in wheat germ, beans, poultry, eggs, cashews, and oysters.

Alcohol lowers testosterone levels. "Alcohol, when consumed excessively for too long," says *Age Erasers for Men*, "can have a direct effect on the testicles, decreasing production of the male hormone testosterone."

Meat is more ambiguous.

Says Barnard, "The high-fat, meat-based diet boosts testosterone's effects." But, according to research from the University of Utah in Salt Lake City, foods high in fat actually lower testosterone.

Given the uncertainties of the research, it's probably safest to go easy on meat consumption.

INSULIN

Most people don't think of insulin as a hormone, but it is.

"Insulin helps the body to metabolize or break down glucose, or blood sugar, in a form that can be utilized by the cells for energy," Mindell says. Originating in the pancreas, a large gland below the stomach, insulin enters the bloodstream when blood glucose (sugar) rises above its normal level.

Over time, the process can easily go bad. "As people age, they are likely to develop insulin resistance," Mindell says. "That is, they cannot use insulin effectively to turn glucose into energy."

Stanford University's Gerald Reaven, M.D., estimates that 25 percent of normal healthy non-diabetic Americans have insulin resistance. Aronne notes that a diet full of simple carbohydrates, starches, and saturated fat can worsen the problem.

Since insulin resistance keeps the body from absorbing glucose, the glucose remains in the bloodstream. *Aging: A Natural History* notes, "The excess glucose in the bloodstream reacts with hemoglobin [red blood cells] in a free radical oxidation." As noted earlier, free radicals can mean trouble.

There is a way out of high glucose levels. As Carper puts it, "To control blood sugar, your body may then dump more insulin in your blood." The extra insulin will change the sugar into a form that the body can use.

So all is well—except that high amounts of insulin stimulate the appetite, increase the body's amount of fat, and encourage high blood pressure, coronary artery diseases, high cholesterol, cancer, and—especially—diabetes.

Mindell defines diabetes as "the inability of the body to metabolize and use foods properly." He adds, "Diabetes can lead to serious complications, including heart disease, kidney disease, stroke, and severe circulatory problems."

But, Mindell notes, "A proper diet and life-style can prevent or delay the onset of diabetes." A low-fat, plant-based diet, adds Barnard, "cuts out fats that interfere with insulin."

Some specific recommendations from the experts:

Chromium-rich foods are beneficial because insufficient chromium can trigger insulin resistance; chromium helps to ensure that the body has the right amounts of insulin and blood sugar. High-chromium foods include whole wheat and other whole grains, broccoli, peanuts, mushrooms, and brewer's yeast.

"Complex carbohydrates, the kind found in legumes and grains," says Mindell, "burn slowly and steadily in the body . . . thus giving the insulin the time it needs to utilize glucose"—and, says Fries, "to clear the sugar from the blood."

Monounsaturated fat such as canola oil and olive oil may control insulin levels. Herbs such as cinnamon, fenugreek, and turmeric stimulate insulin efficiency— "meaning your body gets by with less of the hormone," says Carper. Foods full of vitamin E—including whole grains, wheat germ, sweet potatoes, sunflower oil, kale, brussels sprouts, broccoli, nuts, and beans—may fight insulin resistance. Vegetables may help, too; as Mindell says, "Fiber-rich foods help lower insulin needs."

Fruit is controversial. Most experts recommend it. It's rich in fiber, and Dr. Richard Deeb, author of *Live to Be 100+: Healthy Choices for Maximizing Your Life*, notes that fructose, the sugar in fruit, is very low in glucose, the specific sugar that triggers insulin production. It's so low that, according to Stini, "[fructose] has been frequently recommended for diabetics."

But Carper says that fructose can make the body produce more insulin. "All sugars can equally boost insulin needs," she says.

Although this is an area in which no one yet has a definitive answer, the bulk of the literature leans toward eating fruit.

Despite their disagreements on fruit, the experts do agree on one thing: Keep your sugar intake down. And not just table sugar; baked goods tend to be high in sugar, too.

And, of course, any foods that build fat can trigger diabetes.

OTHER HORMONES

Other hormones, such as melatonin, DHEA, and human growth hormone, are currently available only in supplements or by prescription. Food may not carry or stimulate them. They'll be covered in a later section of this book.

CAFFEINE

Caffeine can weaken bones by preventing them from getting enough calcium. It can deplete the body of B vitamins. It can increase the flow of urination to the point where the body can become dehydrated. It can aggravate prostate problems in some men. It can cause or worsen heart arrhythmia (irregular heartbeat).

What's more, says Barnard, "caffeine is clearly addicting."

CAFFEINE CONTROVERSIES

If it sounds as if caffeine is the devil's brew, be aware that some claims about it are in dispute. For example:

- *Caffeine causes depression.* "Removing refined sugar and caffeine from your diet could be all you need to do to banish depression," advises *Staying Young*. On the other hand, says *Live Longer, Live Better,* caffeine may "in susceptible people prevent depression." If you believe that caffeine in your diet may be changing your mood, check with your doctor.

- *Caffeine raises cholesterol.* To reduce cholesterol, says Ryback, "give up caffeine." But Barnard says that although coffee can raise cholesterol levels, "what determines coffee's effect is not its caffeine but the method of brewing. Caffeine does not raise cholesterol levels, and drip and instant coffee have little or no effect on cholesterol."

The definitive truth on these matters isn't settled yet.

CAFFEINE AND LONGEVITY

Despite caffeine's threats to health, Chopra reveals that most of the people in a 1973 study of 79 people 87 years old and older drank coffee. And a ten-year study of 85,000 women, tracked by the National Institutes of Health, revealed that drinking coffee, caffeinated or not, didn't seem to raise the women's risk of heart disease.

Clearly, caffeine causes more confusion than most of us have ever thought.

Perhaps a sensible approach to the issue of caffeine and longevity comes from Georgakas. While he notes that "caffeine has no positive input in the diet," he also admits, "its consumption in very moderate quantities may not be particularly harmful."

HOW MODERATE IS "VERY MODERATE"?

Most experts recommend no more than three six-ounce cups of coffee per day. Some go lower; for instance, *Age Erasers for Men* allows two five-ounce cups in a day.

"Tolerance for caffeine declines with age . . . [so] you may want to reduce your intake or eliminate it entirely to avoid unpleasant side effects as you grow older," advises *Live Longer, Live Better.*

Lower your caffeine intake gradually. Going cold turkey can bring on withdrawal symptoms such as headache, anxiety, and depression.

As *Age Erasers for Women* explains, quoting Richard Podell, M.D., of the University of Medicine and Dentistry of New Jersey, "No two people are the same. . . . One cup of coffee can cause problems in some [people], and other [people] seem to have a much higher tolerance."

If you find that caffeine affects you strongly, try easing yourself down from your current level of consumption.

SO, WHAT SHOULD YOU EAT?

WHICH FOODS HAVE THE MOST OF THE BEST INGREDIENTS—AND which foods should you shun?

Table 2.1 is a list based on the preceding sections. Eat as many of the "approved" foods as you can. Avoid the "disapproved" foods. And be moderate in eating the ones in the "controversial" column.

The foods noted with an asterisk (*) are the ones that the text mentions most often. They're the best, worst, and most controversial of the foods in the list.

Some foods pop up in two categories, because different ways of preparing them earn different ratings. Chicken, for example, gets a "controversial" rating in its skinless version, while chicken nuggets are to be avoided.

Some foods aren't in any categories, simply because there isn't room for every kind of food. Still, if you don't find a particular food here, you can probably find one like it. Butter, for example, isn't here—but other dairy products are, and you can make your judgment on butter based on the listing for its relatives. Celery isn't here, but other green vegetables are. And so on.

On with the list.

TABLE 2.1   HEALTHY AND UNHEALTHY FOODS

BAKED GOODS (EXCEPT BREADS)

Approved	Controversial	Disapproved
		cakes
		cookies
		muffins

BEVERAGES (EXCEPT DAIRY BEVERAGES)

Approved	Controversial	Disapproved
fruit juices	alcohol*	coffee
water	water (tap)	sodas/soft
(bottled)		drinks*
		tea

DAIRY PRODUCTS

	Approved	Controversial	Disapproved
Cheese		uncreamed cottage	cheddar cheese
		cheese	Swiss cheese
Milk		low-fat milk	ice cream
		nonfat milk	whole milk

FLAVORINGS

	Approved	Controversial	Disapproved
Oils		canola oil	coconut oil
		corn oil*	safflower oil
		fish oil	
		olive oil*	
		sunflower oil	
Sweeteners		honey	brown sugar
			white sugar

FLAVORINGS *continued*

	Approved	Controversial	Disapproved
Other flavorings	basil		margarine*
	capsaicin		salad dressing
	(cayenne)		mayonnaise
	cinnamon		salt*
	fenugreek		sauce mixes
	garlic*		soy sauce
	lemon juice		
	lime juice		
	oregano		
	peppers		
	red peppers		
	turmeric		
	vinegar		

FRUITS AND VEGETABLES

	Approved	Controversial	Disapproved
Fruits	apples*		
	apricots		
	avocados		
	bananas*		
	cantaloupe*		
	figs		
	grapefruit		
	kiwi fruit		
	oranges		
	papaya		
	peaches		
	prunes		
	strawberries		
	watermelon		
Leafy green vegetables	bok choy		
	broccoli*		
	brussels sprouts*		
	collard greens		

continued on next page

TABLE 2.1   HEALTHY AND UNHEALTHY FOODS *continued*

FRUITS AND VEGETABLES *continued*

Approved	Controversial	Disapproved
cabbage*		
cauliflower*		
kale*		
lettuce		
mustard greens		
spinach*		
turnip greens		

Green vegetables

legumes*		
beans*		
soybeans		
lentils*		
peas*		

Yellow and orange vegetables

carrots*		
corn		
popcorn (air-popped)		
potatoes*		
pumpkin		
sweet potatoes*		
yams		

Other vegetables

onions		pickles
red onions		
yellow onions		
shallots		
tomatoes		

GRAINS AND GRAIN PRODUCTS

	Approved	Controversial	Disapproved
Bread	whole-grain bread* whole wheat bread	pasta*	white bread pizza crust

Whole grains

cereals
barley
oats
oat bran
oatmeal*
white rice*
brown rice
wheat
wheat bran
wheat germ*
whole wheat

MEAT

	Approved	Controversial	Disapproved
Beef		beef liver	hamburgers hot dogs pot roast
Pork		bacon	
Lamb			
Poultry		chicken (skinless)* eggs* turkey (skinless)	chicken nuggets

continued on next page

TABLE 2.1   HEALTHY AND UNHEALTHY FOODS *continued*

FISH

	Approved	Controversial	Disapproved
		cod	
		flounder	
		haddock	
		halibut	
		herring	
		mackerel	
		salmon*	
		sardines*	
		sole	
		trout	
		rainbow trout	
		tuna	
Shellfish		clams	
		crab	
		lobster	
		oysters	
		scallops	
		shrimp	

NUTS

	Approved	Controversial	Disapproved
	almonds		
	peanuts*		
	walnuts		

OTHER FOODS

	Approved	Controversial	Disapproved
	brewer's yeast*		candy
	mushrooms		chocolate
			potato chips
			soup/broth

ORGANIC PRODUCE

Organic produce, free of pesticides, preservatives, and chemical fertilizers, tends to rank among the healthiest, most life-prolonging foods available.

Brace yourself before you go shopping. "Organic produce may cost more and look less perfect than what is sold in supermarkets," *Live Longer, Live Better* cautions. "Also, produce that isn't treated with wax and chemicals doesn't stay fresh as long as treated produce, so you will have to shop more often and use up what you buy right away."

"A second option," advises Georgakas, "is to patronize a farmers' market. Small truck farmers usually employ more traditional growing methods, and they can be asked what pesticides they may have used. Very rarely will they wax or color their products."

Organic food is not a cure-all. As Fossel says, "Toxins are included in all food, even those unexposed to pesticides and herbicides."

To be doubly careful, recommends *Live Longer, Live Better*, "scrub fruits and vegetables under cold running water with a vegetable brush just before you plan to use them. . . . Use a little dish-washing detergent, then rinse thoroughly."

VEGETARIANISM

Do vegetarians outlive carnivores? It looks that way.

VEGETARIANISM VERSUS ILLNESS

Vegetarians live five to ten years longer than non-vegetarians. A vegetarian diet can fight cancer, heart disease, high blood pressure, high cholesterol, low immunity, arteriosclerosis, diabetes, and maybe even bad moods. For instance:

- In a study of vegetarians and nonvegetarians at the German Cancer Research Center, the immune systems of the vegetarians had more than double the power to kill cancer cells than those of the nonvegetarians.

- Orlock quotes a study of 6,000 vegetarians and 5,000 nonvegetarians, finding that the "vegetarians [were] significantly less likely to die of cancer or heart disease."

- Arnot says, "Vegetarians naturally eat meals that create extremely even blood sugar levels, which may be why they appear so mellow."

- "Vegetarians have less Type II diabetes, gallstones, kidney stones, [and] osteoporosis," says Carper. "They have much higher levels of plant antioxidants."

- *Staying Young* discloses that Dr. Dean Ornish of the Preventive Medicine Research Institute, a well-respected authority on diet and longevity, "has shown that a vegetarian diet, coupled with exercise and meditation, can dramatically lower blood cholesterol levels and reverse the arteriosclerotic plaques that form the basis for heart disease." Dr. William Roberts, editor-in-chief of the *American Journal of Cardiology*, has said, "If we—that is, society— switched to a vegetarian diet, arteriosclerotic coronary artery disease, which accounts for most heart disease, would vanish."

In sum, vegetarians live healthier than carnivores, and a healthier life is often a longer one.

LIMITATIONS AND VARIETY

Eating vegetarian requires planning. "As with any restricted diet," *Live Longer, Live Better* warns, "a vegan diet [one that avoids all animal products, including dairy and eggs] limited to one or only a few foods can be dangerous." Arnot adds, "In a halfhearted or ill-thought-through effort to be vegetarian, many of us fall flat on our faces. If you eat a mostly vegetarian diet, you need to know how to do it."

Protein

"An objection frequently raised to a vegetarian diet is that it provides insufficient protein," says Georgakas. But Barnard notes, "A vegetarian diet provides plenty of protein without any careful planning, provided it is drawn from a variety of foods."

As noted in the section on protein, a diet that includes corn, soybeans, rice, peas, and oatmeal is likely to provide as much protein as most bodies need.

Zinc

Stini says that a study of Dutch vegetarians revealed low levels of zinc in their diets. Zinc being a longevity mineral, vegetarians should make sure to get enough of it. Fortunately, it's in beans and other legumes.

Iron

Some vegetarians may become deficient in iron. For them, the *Age Erasers* books recommend foods rich in vitamin C, which helps the body to absorb the iron in vegetables. Foods rich in both iron and vitamin C include brussels sprouts, broccoli, and cauliflower.

Vitamin B$_{12}$

The problem mentioned most often in the literature is a lack of vitamin B$_{12}$. The reason: B$_{12}$ comes from animals.

The solution, according to Barnard, is to eat foods that are enriched with B$_{12}$. The *Age Erasers* books note that soy milk can help, too.

A more general solution to all these problems is a simple one. "Eat a variety of plant foods," advises *Live Longer, Live Better*. The greater the variety you eat, the more likely you'll get all the nutrients you need.

100 PERCENT VEGAN OR AN OCCASIONAL BURGER?

Although many experts are strictly in favor of vegetarianism—Barnard, for example, advises flatly, "Eliminate animal products from the diet"— some authorities would loosen things a little.

- Arnot doesn't mind the nonvegetarian life as long as it cuts down on bad food in general. "I'm convinced that the reason [vegetarians] feel so good is that they eat so little processed food, simple sugar, or animal fat. I'm not convinced that they feel any better than nonvegetarians who do the same."

- Moore notes that eating animal food doesn't always mean death. "The second-longest lived nation, Switzerland, has more animal fat in its diet than virtually any country in the world, except Austria, another long-lived nation." (He adds, however, that the nation with the longest-living people is Japan, a country with "a diet very low in saturated fat and other animal products.")

- Carper would permit seafood in an otherwise vegetarian diet: "Eating only plant foods (and seafood) seems to give you the best odds on aging slowly and stretching your life to the maximum."

Nurse and dietitian Suzanne Havala says, "If you can keep your meat intake to a small portion, like a side dish, you're probably all right." She adds that a small amount of dairy—no more than three cups per day or three to four egg yolks a week—can be acceptable.

The consensus seems to be that all-out vegetarianism, if well managed, may be the best way to go—but allowing yourself an occasional slice of lean meat won't kill you.

CALORIC RESTRICTION

In the 1930s, using a simple, inexpensive method, Clive McCay of Cornell University extended the life span beyond its known natural limits. He did so with rats, by restricting their diets.

Says Hayflick, "Feeding rats a diet containing all the necessary vitamins and minerals but low in calories"—about 60 percent less food than rats eat when allowed as much food as they want, according to Chopra—"extended their life span significantly."

"Significantly" in this case means by at least a third. "Translated into human terms," says *Search for Immortality*, "this meant that they reached about 150 years of age."

What's more, the rats were healthy, bright-eyed, vigorous, and apparently youthful for that long span. UCLA's Walford says, "The development of a wide variety of cancers was inhibited . . . and beneficial effects on vascular and kidney disease also accrued."

"McCay's experiment has now been performed on many other animals, including fish, mice, silkworms, spiders, fruit flies, rotifers, and daphnia (the last two are microscopic pond animals)," says Hayflick. "The results with all these species have been the same: caloric restriction produced animals with greater longevity." Chopra puts it more boldly: "McCay's method of 'under-nutrition' . . . is the only proven way to extend the maximum life span."

No one knows why. There are many theories as to the cause—slower metabolism in caloric-restricted animals, lower body temperature, and any number of other things—but nothing is conclusive or has been proven.

Can caloric restriction extend human life? No one has done long-term under-nutrition experiments on human longevity. But there is some intriguing anecdotal evidence.

- "The major characteristic of the diet of longevous people is low caloric intake throughout life," says Georgakas, who's studied long-lived people from all over the world.

- Moore notes, "Reducing calorie intake lowers blood pressure, serum cholesterol, and blood sugar levels."

- "Three studies on nonhuman primates (primarily rhesus monkeys) are in progress. The available results suggest that [caloric restriction] can be safely carried out in primates," say Rajindar Sohal of Southern Methodist University's Biological Sciences Department and Richard Weindruch of the University of Wisconsin's Department of Medicine, writing in the journal *Science*.

- The longest-lived people in the world have a calorically light diet. The Japanese, who have a diet that's thin on high-calorie foods such as beef, live longer than other people. The people of Okinawa Island—who, according to Orlock, "consume on average 30 percent fewer calories than other Japanese"—live even longer than other Japanese. As Walford puts it, "Okinawa has 5 to 40 times the incidence of people over 100 years of age as any other Japanese island."

(Promising though it seems, the Okinawa story is inconclusive. Other factors, from genetics to exercise, may contribute to longevity of the Okinawans.)

Anorexics, of course, restrict caloric intake. Are they expected to live long?

No. They go too far in restricting their calories. More importantly, they restrict everything, including the low-fat, high-nutrient, high-fiber foods (fruits and vegetables, for example) that can keep the body running well without adding a lot of calories. Besides, their emotional state—wracked with anxiety—isn't conducive to long life.

Besides anorexics and animals, the most famous test case of caloric restriction is UCLA biogerontologist Roy Walford. Walford, who recommends caloric restriction to lower the risk of cancer, heart disease, arteriosclerosis, and high blood pressure, has been living on a calorie-restricted diet since 1987. He's now in his early 70s. If he's still alive 50 years from now, he'll know that he was right.

To do as he does, Walford says, "Try about a 20 percent restriction, and see how it goes." He defines a 20 percent restriction as "still eating 80 percent of what you would be eating under your usual circumstances . . . [and] 20 percent is only safe if you are very careful about [eating] quality food."

Walford adds that "more [restriction] is too much, unless you are under very close medical supervision." And no matter how much you cut back, he says, do it gradually.

Moreover, Orlock warns, "caloric restriction . . . is not for everyone." It's wrong for children and for women who want to become pregnant.

Not every expert agrees that caloric restriction can be beneficial. For example, Barnard says, "Your metabolic rate can drop to 15 to 20 percent below normal, all as a result of a calorie-restricted diet. And dieters know it. They begin to feel cold, constipated, and out of sorts. Their bodies are literally shutting down biological functions."

But Barnard is in the minority. Although there is no proof that caloric restriction can extend healthy human life, many experts consider it a definite possibility. In fact, the National Institute on Aging has funded caloric-restriction research since the late 1980s, according to the journal *Science News*.

With all this experimention, the research on humans has been done primarily on one person—Walford, experimenting with his own life. As Hayflick puts it, "Walford deserves enormous credit for doing what few humans have attempted, and those of us who know of his efforts to increase our knowledge of human aging wish him well."

MEALS

"The standard American meal," writes Bortz in *Dare to Be 100*, "consists of a cup of coffee for breakfast, a sandwich and a soda for lunch, and then a mound of food for dinner. This gorging meal pattern would do a lion proud, but is it for you?"

Probably not.

- Bortz says, "If you dump the majority of your calories into your system at one time of day, you impose a heavy instantaneous metabolic burden. Your digestive enzymes and hormones, particularly insulin, have a lot of major work to do in a short time interval." Moreover, he says, "A gorging meal pattern raises cholesterol levels."

- Ford agrees: "A two-year study by Allen B. Nicholls of 4,057 men aged 20 and over at the University of Michigan concluded that eating large meals can be as life-shortening as eating a diet high in fat."

- *Age Erasers for Men* notes, "The body can metabolize only so much food at one time, so the excess is likely to become fat."

GRAZING AND MULTIPLE MEALS

A better way is to spread meals throughout the day, or even to graze and nibble instead of taking full meals.

- In April 1996, *Sports Afield* magazine's Michael Segell wrote, "According to new findings published in the *American Journal of Clinical Nutrition,* a six- or nine-meal-a-day diet can lower insulin levels and blood cholesterol and help maintain healthy body weight."

- What's more, grazing can prevent overeating. James Kenney, R.D., Ph.D., a nutrition research specialist says, "If you graze on low-fat, high-fiber foods that aren't packed with calories, such as carrots, apples, peaches, oranges, and red peppers, you'll keep your appetite down."

HOW MANY MEALS?

A rough consensus of the experts recommends four to nine feedings per day, either as small meals or as a mixture of small meals and healthy snacks.

Not that you absolutely must give up three meals a day if you like that pattern or can't escape it. For example, Georgakas says, "There is no evidence that a limited number of regular meals is harmful. The three-major-meals-a-day pattern, which is based on the economic organization of modern society, is acceptable."

But even authorities who approve of that pattern are just as willing to accept more. H. Winter Griffith, M.D., in his *Complete Guide to Symptoms, Illness & Surgery for People over 50,* issues the succinct command, "Eat three meals a day"—but, he adds, "If you get hungry between meals . . . eat fruit, vegetables, or whole-grain snacks."

Thus the rules about the number of meals per day aren't cast in steel—although in general, more and smaller is better than fewer and bigger.

SPACING AND TIMING

Food is like comedy—timing is important. The experts recommend eating on a regular schedule, with meals spaced evenly over the day. As Griffith says, "Regular meals keep the metabolic and digestive systems functioning at their most efficient levels."

"It is very important not to miss a meal," Aronne adds. "If you want a snack at midday, enjoy a healthy one. If you overindulge at one meal—and almost everyone does from time to time—don't skip the next meal. Likewise, don't deliberately miss a meal in order to overeat later." Overeating, he says, overburdens the body.

One meal needs particular mention. Your mother may have been right; it could be the most important meal of the day.

BREAKFAST

Everyone should eat breakfast. And although no meal should be huge, breakfast should be the day's biggest meal. As Georgakas puts it, "Eat breakfast like a lion, lunch like a squirrel, and dinner like a bird."

Why?

Arnot says, "Food has its biggest benefit at breakfast. It wakes up the body and increases metabolism." A souped-up metabolism burns calories fast, which reduces the chance that food will end up as fat.

Ignoring breakfast, on the other hand, can be dangerous.

- Ford says, "At least one study has shown that skipping breakfast increases by 2.5 times the risk of formation of a blood clot that may cause a heart attack or stroke."

- "Skipping breakfast is like running your car when it's low on oil and coolant: It may work, but it's tough on the engine," says *Staying Young*. "Not only is your body starved for fuel in the morning (whether you feel hungry or not), but you're more likely to overeat and grab the wrong foods when you do settle down for a meal."

Virtually all experts recommend whole grains for breakfast, preferably in cereals. Other heavily approved ways to serve whole grains include pancakes, oatmeal, and breads such as muffins and French toast.

Fruit and fruit juice get much approval. Some experts, especially those who are not strict vegetarians, allow a small amount of margarine (up to half a tablespoon per day), skim milk (up to one cup), and egg whites (up to four).

If this breakfast has you feeling hungry later in the day, Aronne recommends, "you may want to eat your first meal a little later in the morning and delay lunch until midafternoon."

But always eat your breakfast. Your mother would want you to, and now she's got a phalanx of doctors behind her.

FOOD PREPARATION

The way you prepare food can be as important as the foods themselves. Preparation can add or withdraw antioxidants, nutrients, and toxins.

Among the methods most often mentioned by longevity experts are the following:

RAW

One of the best ways to prepare food is to prepare it as little as possible.

Georgakas explains, "Raw foods . . . cause minimal strain on the body, as they take only 18 to 24 hours to go through the entire digestive process from ingestion to evacuation. Cooked and processed foods need from 8 to 100 hours to accomplish the same journey and may give off poisons while languishing for long periods in the lower intestinal tract."

What's more, *Age Erasers for Women* says, "cooking food draws out or destroys many vitamins and minerals." (For example, Barnard says, raw vegetables and fruits retain more vitamin C than if they're heavily cooked.)

Some foods aren't eaten raw, of course—chicken, for example. If you want to cook, here are notes about some of the best-known methods.

STEAMING

Many experts recommend steaming. Steamed vegetables are a tasty healthy dish that restaurants happily provide. At home, says Barnard, "Using a collapsible steamer rack, cook vegetables above a small amount of boiling water in a covered pan. This protects nutrients and flavor."

Even Georgakas, who isn't a fan of any kind of cooking—he believes that the most nutritious way to eat many foods is raw—recommends steaming for foods that are inedible uncooked. "Food that must be prepared or softened will suffer the least nutritional loss if steamed," he says.

Georgakas finds an additional benefit. "The broth left over from steaming . . . can be consumed as a soup."

BAKING

Baking is another relatively safe way to cook—depending on how you do it.

To bake safely, Walford says, "(1) start out with wholesome ingredients, meaning whole, unrefined, unprocessed grains, flours, etc.; and (2) . . . reduce the fat/oil content and the sugar content of all of your baking recipes." (Walford warns, though, that "few brand-name baking mixes contain whole-grain flours, so we don't recommend using them often.")

Baked goods from stores or restaurants can cause trouble. Commercial bakeries often make cookies, cakes, doughnuts, pastries, crackers, and pies with trans fats and saturated fat.

Still, some commercial baked goods draw applause from the experts. Baked beans (especially vegetarian baked beans) get high marks from

Barnard for their generous load of fiber. "A baked potato, spared a butter-and-salt bath, is extremely nutritious and easy to digest," says Georgakas.

If it's simple, vegetarian, and low in fat, it's probably healthy when baked.

BROILING

Broiling is another good way to cook. Not only is it relatively healthy, but Walford says, "broiled vegetables are quick and easy to prepare, and can accompany most any main dish elegantly."

Meats, though, are somewhat controversial. Although Aronne finds broiling meat acceptable, Carper says, "Restrict grilled, fried, and broiled meat." She contends that broiled meats can damage arteries.

How to resolve this contradiction? Avoid broiled meats; doing so can't hurt and may help. After all, it's good to cut down on meats in the first place.

FRYING

"The form of cooking to be avoided most is frying," says Georgakas.

"Throw the deep fryer away," recommends *Age Erasers for Men*.

"Totally shun all fried foods," says Ford.

"Avoid foods that are fried," advises Willix.

"Don't fry," pleads Bortz.

Why?

"Vital elements like enzymes [proteins that help biological reactions happen] are destroyed by frying, and the food is made more difficult to digest, placing extra burdens on all parts of the digestive system," says Georgakas.

But more important is fat. When you fry foods, the oils in which they fry permeate them, filling the foods with fat.

Frying adds so much fat that even low-fat foods become fattier than high-fat foods. "Many excellent foods, such as the potato, become anti-longevous when turned into French fries or potato chips," says Georgakas.

Or take the chicken-beef paradox. Ordinarily, a quarter pound of chicken has 27 grams less fat than a quarter pound of cooked, lean beef chuck, according to *Live Longer, Live Better*. But the U.S. Department of Agriculture notes that a fast-food version of a breaded fried chicken sandwich has *more* fat than a quarter-pound hamburger.

The only kind of frying that any expert recommends is dry frying, also known as frying vegetables in their own juices.

To dry fry, Walford recommends that you get a good nonstick skillet and "spray the skillet lightly with olive oil or add a teaspoon of broth, wine, or water before placing [the skillet] over the heat. Once the vegetables have been added, cover the skillet for a minute to discourage liquids from evaporating too quickly. Then, with a rubber spatula or wooden spoon, as the vegetables begin to stick to the pan, stir the brown bits from the bottom of the pan. . . . Add liquids sparingly as you cook the vegetables. To keep them from scorching, cover the skillet and stir frequently."

But other than that—don't fry.

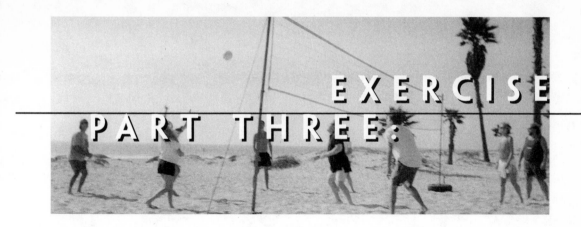

EXERCISE

PART THREE:

- "Perhaps the single most important item in the longevity agenda." That's how author Dan Georgakas describes exercise in *The Methuselah Factors*.

- "If there's anything close to a genuine youth drug, it's sweat," says *Age Erasers for Women*.

- "A moderate and consistent exercise program is all it takes to live longer, live stronger, and live better," writes Earl Mindell in *Earl Mindell's Anti-Aging Bible*.

Exercise can even help the body benefit from diet and other contributors to longevity. "Exercise, in fact, will minimize the need for special diets, supplements, and medications," says Georgakas. Strategies to prevent aging, writes Richard Deeb in *Live to Be 100+*, "are only half as effective without the inclusion of exercise."

Here's the proof:

- "Strenuous physical activity throughout the course of life is the most common thread in the biographies of longevous people," says Georgakas. He notes, "In a survey completed in the 1960s of 402 Americans over age 95, these nonagenarians . . . enjoyed plenty of physical exercise."

- *Sports Afield* magazine fitness and health columnist Michael Segell writes, "In an eight-year study of more than 25,000 obese men at the Cooper Institute for Aerobics Research in Dallas, those who were moderately or very fit had a 70 percent lower mortality rate than the unfit."

- Mindell notes, "A recent study of 10,000 Harvard graduates ages 45 to 84 showed that those who participated in moderately vigorous activities (such as tennis, swimming, jogging, and brisk walking) had up to a 29 percent lower death rate than the sedentary men."

- Mindell mentions a study in which "men who began exercising late in life (after age 65) lived up to six months longer than couch potatoes."

- An American Cancer Society survey of over a million people found that exercising lowered death rates from every major disease. "A Finnish study discovered that woodcutters live seven to eight years longer than office workers," Georgakas reveals. "An inactive life-style . . . contributes to about 250,000 deaths annually," reports heart doctor Robert Willix in *Healthy at 100*. In a Stanford University study, men who didn't exercise had a 23 percent higher risk of death than men who did.

On and on the statistics go, demonstrating that exercise can add years to one's life.

That wasn't always the conventional wisdom. "Until the nineteenth century," says Hayflick in *How and Why We Age*, "there was still a widespread belief that vigorous exercise was harmful to the body and reduced longevity." "Until about 1960, medicine warned older people away from any exercise more strenuous than walking," writes Orlock in *The End of Aging*. "Supposedly, vigorous activity would wear out the body's machine."

There were exceptions. In the thirteenth century, Oxford scholar Roger Bacon studied longevity and concluded that the neglect of exercise (among other things) shortened life.

That's the consensus today. And yet . . .

THE CASE AGAINST EXERCISE

If the human body's maximum life span is 115 to 120 years, no amount of exercise can make it last to 125.

As Orlock says: "Becoming an 80-year-old Olympian may not necessarily add years to one's life. . . . While maintaining peak strength, exceptional stamina, and robust appearance may feel good, these payoffs may make no difference in actual life span."

What's more, exercise may not help people even rise toward the maximum.

- "There is no good evidence that life expectation is increased in physically active older people," Hayflick says. "If it were, we would expect to find that all, or most, of our oldest people are, or were, physically active, and this is not true. Most, in fact, are sedentary."

- "If exercise did increase longevity," Hayflick adds, "we would find lumberjacks, stevedores, and baseball players outliving taxicab drivers, sedentary businessmen, and general loafers. This does not seem to be the case." In fact, Georgakas says, "As a group, male professional athletes have life spans below the national averages."

- Even if exercise may be good for you, too much exercise may not. A study in the *Journal of the American Medical Association* researched people at different levels of fitness. Although the unfit people died younger than the moderately fit, so did the very fit.

- Hayflick debunks studies showing that athletes live longer than other people by noting that the athletes live not very much longer. In fact, he says, athletes spent so much time exercising and gained so few extra years that "the years they gained were . . . spent jogging!"

RESOLVING THE CONTRADICTIONS

"Exercise may increase longevity," Hayflick admits, but "only to the extent that it modifies disease processes."

And on that contention, almost every expert agrees. "Studies show that exercise cuts the risk of life-threatening diseases," says *Live Longer, Live Better*. As Orlock says, "Conditions that can improve with regular rigorous activity provide a laundry list of just about everything that can go wrong as we age."

For example:

- Exercise can improve heart performance. Says Peter Wood, Ph.D., of Stanford University's Center for Research in Disease Prevention, "With regular exercise, the heart becomes a more efficient pump."

- Exercise can decrease the chance of death by stroke. "In a 22-year [study] of more than 5,300 Japanese Americans," says Mindell, "researchers found a strong association between a sedentary lifestyle and an increased risk of stroke."

- Exercise can help to prevent cancer and slow the growth of existing cancerous tumors. *Age Erasers for Men* reports a study in which "men who expended at least 1,000 calories a week (walking up one flight of stairs daily expends about 28 calories per week) were up to 50 percent less likely than sedentary men to develop colon cancer." In *Eat Right, Live Longer,* Barnard writes, "Researchers at the University of Southern California found that one to three hours of exercise per week during the reproductive years cuts breast cancer risk by 30 percent."

- Exercise can help the brain think clearly, solve problems, recall memories, be alert, and reason accurately. A study involving researchers from Harvard, Yale, Duke, Brandeis, and Mt. Sinai School of Medicine examined almost 1,200 fit people in their 70s and found that exercise kept their minds healthy, active, and sharp. Exactly how is not fully known, but some authorities suspect that exercise may stimulate the flow of blood into the brain.

- Exercise can reduce stress. *Live Longer, Live Better* says, "In one study, physically active people who were asked to solve a series of unsolvable problems suffered less stress striving to do so than did an inactive control group."

- Exercise can enlarge the arteries and slow down the speed at which they stiffen up, thus fighting off atherosclerosis.

- Exercise can empower the immune system. The *Age Erasers* books testify that exercise "strengthens the vigilance of the immune system by increasing circulation of antibodies in the blood."

- And exercise can prevent or forestall diabetes—but the *Age Erasers* books warn diabetics to exercise with care because improper exercise can cause fatigue, confusion, headache, palpitations, shakiness, profuse sweat, or dizziness.

So even though exercise is no *guarantee* of longer life, the consensus agrees with Stanford's Bortz, who writes in *Dare to Be 100*: "A walk to the store, library, or post office is better medicine than anything I have in my black bag."

What about Hayflick's point that you'll spend—or waste—your extra years of life exercising?

Some people enjoy exercise, or at least the benefits that it brings. For them, the time spent exercising is no waste at all, but a pleasure.

If you're not one of those people, then *carpe vitam*—enjoy the years that you have, because they may be fewer than those of the people who exercise.

EXERCISE MYTHS, LEGENDS, AND LIES

IT'S DANGEROUS TO EXERCISE WHEN YOU'RE OLD

"It's never too late to get in shape," Cornell University's Aronne writes in *Weigh Less, Live Longer*. According to the *Age Erasers* volumes, "Even if you're a little late getting started, you can still benefit from exercise."

- Says John J. Medina, Ph.D., of the University of Washington School of Medicine and author of *The Clock of Ages: Why We Age—How We Age—Winding Back the Clock*, "One study conducted in 69 to 74-year-old men suggests that gains up to 22 percent in strength (compared to pre-training achievement) can occur even if the older adult was previously sedentary."

- Hayflick adds that exercise can rescue even those conditions that deteriorate with age: "We can improve cardiac efficiency, pulmonary function, and bone calcium levels."

- In a 1997 issue of the *Journal of the American Medical Association*, Lawrence Kushi, Ph.D., of the University of Minnesota School of Public Health announced the results of a seven-year study of more than 40,000 postmenopausal women. The women who exercised four times a week had a death rate one-third lower than the women who didn't exercise.

So is exercising dangerous? Not nearly as dangerous as not exercising.

NO PAIN, NO GAIN

"The 'no pain, no gain' approach to exercise is not necessary and can even be harmful in some cases," says Deeb.

"The phrase 'no pain, no gain' has been retranslated to 'less pain, more gain,'" Bortz says. "As with most things, moderation seems best."

Not that even moderate exercise is necessarily a snap. *Dr. Bob Arnot's Guide to Turning Back the Clock* concedes, "When you begin, every motion seems painful." "Some muscle soreness and stiffness is natural after exercise, particularly if it is more than usual exertion," Bortz explains.

Fortunately, Bortz goes on, "the aches are minor, disappear after a few minutes, and are actually an integral part of becoming better conditioned." What's more, Arnot says, "the better you get, the less exertion you perceive."

What if you do find pain (or, rather, it finds you)?

As Arnot says, "Back off when it hurts"—but don't stop exercising altogether; just proceed more carefully. After you exercise, do a cool-down (explained later on), which "helps you avoid some of the muscle tightening and soreness that can accompany exercise," says Aronne. Bortz adds, "Ice and anti-inflammatory medicines help shorten the recovery from pain."

No exercise program can avoid pain altogether. As Stanford's Fries writes in *Living Well*, "Exercise programs always have setbacks in which there are periods of increased pain."

Which brings us to our next subject . . .

EXERCISE CAN INJURE YOU

This one's no myth. "Every person without exception who lives an active life will have injuries," Bortz says. Fries notes, "Most people starting exercise programs have two or three minor injuries in the first year."

To reduce the risk of injury, get protective gear. The *Age Erasers* books suggest "padding on knees, elbows, and other likely trouble spots."

Proper warm-ups and cool-downs, as described below, can alleviate these problems. So can drinking plenty of fluids or applying heat or massage to the hurt area. See a doctor "if you have bleeding, intense pain, numbness, severely restricted movement, or swelling that doesn't abate in a few hours," advises *Live Longer*.

If all else fails, Fries says, "substitute another activity for the one you are having trouble with and thus maintain your fitness program. Sometimes you cannot, and you just have to lay off for a while."

Finally, don't worry too much about injuries. Getting in shape makes them less likely. A Tufts University study put a nursing home's frailest residents on a weight-training program. In two months, their muscles had tripled their strength, their coordination and sense of balance grew—thereby, in all probability, reducing the likelihood of falling and getting hurt.

YOU DON'T NEED TO EXERCISE
EARLIER IN LIFE

Sorry. *Age Erasers for Women*, citing a British study, puts it clearly: "The sooner you start exercising, the better. Women who started exercising between ages 15 and 25 had a 63 percent reduction in their risk for stroke [compared to women who didn't exercise when young]." *Age Erasers for Men* adds, "Guys who started regularly exercising between ages 15 and 25 had 70 percent less risk of stroke than nonexercisers."

So the best advice on exercise comes in two words: Start now.

EXERCISE WIPES OUT BAD FOOD

No, it doesn't. Says Walford, "Avoid the myth that exercise is a sort of universal panacea for health problems, and especially the idea that it's okay to have a high-calorie, even slightly junky diet, as long as you burn off those extra calories by exercise. That's not the case." As Barnard says, "Physical activity works *with* a healthy diet; it cannot replace it."

Fortunately, Barnard adds, "Physical activity makes your appetite more regular and predictable. Binges are far less likely." In other words, exercise helps the body eat in a healthy way.

YOU NEED A GYM
FOR A PROPER WORKOUT

No, you don't. "You can get the exercise you need by walking around a park or shopping mall, dancing at a nightclub, playing tennis, or anything else that simply gets your body moving," says Barnard.

Whether you exercise at a gym or at home, warns *Live Longer, Live Better*, "never exercise on a nonresilient floor (concrete or tile, for example), even if it is carpeted. A hard floor won't absorb impact and is likely to cause injuries."

EXERCISE CAN KILL YOU

This one has some truth.

"Every winter, people will die from the exertion of shoveling snow, and every summer a fair percentage of tennis players and golfers become victims of heart attack and heatstroke," Georgakas admits. "In the United States, many high school athletes will develop degenerative diseases by midlife. . . . Physical exercise, perhaps the single most important item in the longevity agenda, can be a cruel double-edged sword."

What is going on here?

In his book *Human Aging*, Salisbury State University's DiGiovanna explains, "Very strenuous activities present a special danger to those with arteriosclerosis because people tend to hold their breath while pulling or pushing with great force. Blood pressure rises to a very high level during such maneuvers, placing a great burden on the heart and arteries. A heart attack, a stroke, or damage to the retina or vitreous humor [in the eye] can result."

You can prevent these problems by "minimizing exercises requiring great strength and maximizing activities involving free movement of parts of the body," DiGiovanna advises.

And by simply being sensible. "Moderate but not excessive exercise appears best from the health standpoint," Walford says.

Finally—and fortunately—deaths from exercise are rare. "There is one death per 18,000 exercisers per year," Bortz reports.

So don't avoid exercise. Although it can kill you, it probably won't. Not exercising is likelier to kill you than exercising is.

"IF YOU FEEL A LITTLE RELUCTANCE TO GET ON YOUR FEET, DON'T worry," Barnard says. "That is simply a clue that you, like all heavenly bodies, obey the laws of nature"—specifically, the law that bodies at rest tend to stay at rest.

A way to get around this problem, says Bortz, is to "collect information about the active life-style." He explains, "The more you learn, the more you will identify how this critical commitment will benefit every one of the rest of your days."

Here's some information and advice that may help.

GET A CHECKUP

"Your physician," says Bortz, "should be an active ally in your [exercise] effort." "An undiagnosed health problem can make exercise dangerous, even life-threatening in rare cases," advises *Live Longer, Live Better*.

A pre-exercise checkup is especially necessary for anyone who is:

diabetic;

over 35;

a smoker;

overweight;

living a sedentary life;

regularly using any medication, especially one that affects heart rate, such as beta blockers;

or living with a history of a heart-related problem—for instance, high blood pressure, irregular heartbeat, high cholesterol levels, stroke, or angina.

HAVE FUN

"The key to making [exercise] a regular habit is to find an activity you enjoy," Aronne says. Georgakas advises, "Prolongevous exercises . . . should be movements [that] the individual enjoys, sees as valuable, and finds easy."

In addition to exercise that itself is enjoyable, you can do other things while exercising—listening to music or watching television—that are fun as well.

The most popular ways to enjoy yourself while exercising follow:

GET PARTNERS

Bortz recommends, "Find other people like you who are active. Find out how they started and what keeps them going."

"Exercising with a friend, or with a small group of people at a similar level, can be an excellent way to stay in the exercise habit," Aronne advises. "Hopefully your family will participate as well," Bortz adds.

Besides, exercising solo can be boring. Exercising with someone else offers the chance to chat or to compete (if you *want* to compete, that is).

HAVE GOALS

"Set short-term goals with measurable results," recommends *Live Longer, Live Better*. "When you reach [a] goal, give yourself a small nonfood reward . . . for your accomplishment," Aronne says. David Ryback, in his book *Look Ten Years Younger, Live Ten Years Longer*, suggests making the reward "something you enjoy but wouldn't ordinarily give yourself."

"Then set a new goal immediately," Aronne concludes. DiGiovanna says, "The intensity or duration of each exercise or the frequency with which it is performed each week should be increased gradually."

In addition to short-term goals, set long-term ones. To pick a goal, Aronne says, "Imagine a physical activity you have always wanted to do."

Running a marathon, climbing a mountain, carrying your bride over the threshold, or lifting more weight than that show-off at the gym—all are strong goals. Then pick a date, months away, to reach the goal.

Another kind of long-term goal is based on your body's needs. Different exercises affect different bodily conditions.

For example, Ford (in his book *18 Natural Ways to Look and Feel Half Your Age*) says that osteoporosis can be fought by "brisk walking or jogging for at least 30 minutes four times a week with 45 minutes of strength-building exercises on alternate days." To reverse heart disease, Barnard recommends "a half-hour walk each day or an hour three times a week." Check with your doctor on the best exercises for your particular body.

WRITE IT DOWN

"Keeping an exercise log allows you to monitor your routine and keep an eye out for obstacles and barriers," Aronne advises. "For example, you may discover that it is harder for you to exercise regularly under stress."

A written record of your exercising can provide a positive experience, too. As *Live Longer, Live Better* says, "Seeing progress on a weekly chart will motivate you."

GO SLOW

When you begin an exercise program, go easy on both the strength and the length of the workout. "The worst thing you can do is try too hard initially and burn yourself out before allowing your form of exercise to become a habit," Ryback says.

A good exercise for starting out is plain old walking, but any exercise that you enjoy will do if you go at it lightly.

"A SLOW STEADY REGULAR EXERCISE PROGRAM IS ONE OF THE SAFEST and surest ways of daring to be 100," says Bortz. True enough; but figuring out how often, for how long, and at what time to exercise isn't always easy.

THE MINIMUM AND THE OPTIMUM

Mayo Clinic cardiologist Thomas Kottke says, "The population, on the average, is so sedentary that any exercise other than changing TV channels or cracking a beer is great."

His is a minority view. Most experts recommend that for any health improvement, exercise at least three times per week at a minimum of 20 minutes per exercise session.

At least and *at a minimum* are the key phrases for that schedule. Even better, according to authorities with the U.S. Centers for Disease Control, the American Geriatrics Society, and the Institute of Aerobics Research, is to do about half an hour, every day if you can manage it—although skipping a day from time to time is no big deal.

What about more exercise—say, an hour a day? It may be helpful, but it's unnecessary and may even be harmful.

Walford says, "The positive health benefits of exercise increase rapidly up to a certain point—corresponding to about 15 miles of jogging per week (three hours of jogging)—and then plateau out."

Walford and others add that free radical damage can result from overdoing it: the body takes in more oxygen than its cells can handle. As Bortz warns, "Over-training not only fails to increase resistance to infection, but it also probably lowers it."

So keep the training moderate.

HOW SOON AFTER EATING
SHOULD YOU EXERCISE?

The experts disagree. Their advice ranges from exercising immediately after meals to waiting a few hours.

Since there is no strong consensus, try exercising at different times to find the time that works best for you.

And once you find that time . . .

BE REGULAR

"Most long-living people incorporate strenuous activities into their habitual routines to the highest degree possible," says Georgakas.

After all, as Ryback says, doing exercise as part of the regular daily routine "will help make it a permanent fixture in your life." Georgakas explains, "Scattering prolongevous activities throughout the daily and weekly schedule is the surest way of getting up to a daily average that can be maintained for a lifetime."

Although getting onto a regular exercise schedule is a good thing to do, don't get worried if you slip a little from time to time. Like other anxieties, stressing out over exercise schedules doesn't contribute to longevity.

FOR HOW MANY WEEKS OR MONTHS
SHOULD YOU EXERCISE?

There is no limit.

As Georgakas says, "The major ingredients for unusual life spans appear to [include] . . . a lifelong history of physical activity." "Exercise programs lasting only a few weeks produce little benefit," adds DiGiovanna.

If you quit, your body can revert to the shape that it had before you began to exercise. For example, says DiGiovanna, an exercise program can raise the heart's ability to pump blood and the endocrine system's power to combat diabetes; but, he warns, "this rise begins to be reversed within days of ending the exercise program."

In other words, don't quit. Occasional breaks are okay, but never give up completely.

WARM-UP, COOL-DOWN, AND VARIATIONS

WARMING UP

Always warm up. "Any athlete knows that you don't just hurl your body from rest into exercise," advises Willix.

Why?

- "Muscles don't deliver as much energy unless they are run at a higher-than-resting-state temperature," Arnot explains.

- *Staying Young* says that a warm-up "prepare[s] your . . . respiratory system for your workout."

- Arnot adds, "If you start without a warm-up, you may cause an irregular heart rhythm."

The warm-up should last about five to ten minutes. Many authorities recommend such gentle activities as walking, stretching, doing a leisurely version of the workout proper, and combinations of all three.

COOLING DOWN

Don't quit your workout instantly. "Suddenly stopping a high-energy activity without a cool-down causes blood to pool in the muscles you have been using, which can cause dizziness as well as [subsequent] pain, swelling, and stiffness," *Live Longer, Live Better* explains. "Cool-down also helps the body remove waste products created during a workout."

To cool down, do as you did during warm-up: walking, stretching, and/or easy versions of the main exercise.

VARYING THE WORKOUT

Don't do the same exercises all the time. "Too much repetition can strain muscles and increase your risk of injury. It can also make exercise sessions monotonous," says *Live Longer, Live Better*.

Mixing and matching exercises is called cross-training. "Popular cross-training combinations are walking or jogging, cycling, and swimming, which complement each other well," recommends *Live Longer, Live Better*.

But, *Age Erasers for Men* warns, if you take up a new sport, ease into it slowly. "Work at gradually increasing the strength and flexibility of the muscles you'll be using."

SPECIFIC EXERCISES

THE EXPERTS RECOMMEND FOUR DIFFERENT KINDS OF EXERCISES: aerobic exercise, strength building, stretching, and physical activities that aren't conventionally considered exercises.

AEROBIC EXERCISE

Aerobics isn't all Lycra leotards, loud Muzak at 120 beats per minute, and videotapes by celebrities so bright and cheery that you want to slap them silly. (Thank God.)

"Aerobic exercise is the brisk rhythmic movement we use when we walk, jog, swim, bicycle, cross-country ski, or when we play demanding sports like soccer, hockey, basketball, or fast singles tennis," explains Ford. *Live Longer, Live Better* adds, "Any exercise consisting of rhythmic, continuous movement that utilizes the large muscle groups of the body is fair game."

"These exercises enable us to restore the youthfulness of our heart, lungs, and arteries and to maintain them at the same healthy level for the rest of our lives," says Ford.

University of South Carolina professor of family medicine William Simpson, quoted in the *Age Erasers* books, has put it forcefully: "If there were ever a fountain of youth, this is it."

WEIGHT-BEARING EXERCISE

The best aerobic exercise is weight-bearing. Weight-bearing exercise involves "your feet hitting the ground with at least the impact that brisk walking produces," says *Age Erasers for Men*. Walking, tennis, and dancing are weight-bearing exercises.

Not all aerobic exercise is weight-bearing. Swimming and cycling, for instance, don't involve your feet hitting the ground. Nonetheless, they are still good exercises, as will be seen on upcoming pages. In fact, any aerobic exercise can provide benefits.

HOW AEROBICS WORKS

Aerobics can help to extend your life in numerous areas. Among them:

- The heart. Ford offers a startling statistic: "Studies have shown that a healthy 90-year-old heart can pump just as effectively as the heart of a 20-year-old. But this is only true if the 90-year-old heart has been maintained in good condition by regular aerobic exercise."

- Blood vessels. "Exercise, if it is to prevent arteriosclerosis, needs to be aerobic or endurance in type," says Fries in *Living Well*. As the University of South Carolina's Simpson says, "Exercise tends to dilate [blood] vessels so that the heart can pump more easily to supply blood to the rest of the body."

- Stroke. "[Blood] clots are the principal cause of strokes, and exercise increases the clot-dissolving factors in the blood," explains *Staying Young*.

- Stress. *Age Erasers for Women* quotes University of Kansas psychologist David Holmes: "Regular aerobic workouts reduce stress more effectively than meditation, psychiatric intervention, biofeedback, and conventional stress management."

  Live Longer, Live Better says, "Aerobic workouts trigger the release of hormones in the brain that lessen anxiety and offset depression." *Staying Young* isn't as certain but offers this view: "Whether it's the increased blood flow to the brain, the release of endorphins and other feel-good hormones, the discharge of hostility, some reduction of emotional strain, or all of the above, a regular program of aerobic exercise can improve your mood and raise your morale."

- Diabetes. "Aerobic exercise," says *Staying Young*, "may prevent people . . . from becoming diabetic."

  How? Working muscles need glucose, so aerobic exercise pulls glucose from the bloodstream into the muscle cells. Insulin helps those cells use the glucose. "Regular aerobic exercise makes [muscle] cells more receptive to insulin" (to quote the *Age Erasers* books)—and as a consequence, the body needs to produce less insulin to help the muscles. And a body that's producing less insulin is a body less likely to get diabetes.

- The brain. Ford says, "A regular program of aerobic exercise can benefit the mind, specifically by enhancing memory recall, response and reaction time, mental agility, and overall cognitive function." Dr. Joanne Stevenson, a nursing professor at Ohio State University, has said, "Real quick thinking and real quick gaining of ideas— getting the whole gestalt—slows down through middle adulthood and into old age. Aerobic exercise would slow down this slowdown."

- Lungs. *Age Erasers for Women* advises, "An aerobic exercise program . . . will help keep your lungs functioning at peak efficiency."

"One recent study of men and women in their sixties showed that their cardiorespiratory function improved 25 to 30 percent during 12 months of regular, moderate aerobic activity," notes *Live Longer, Live Better*.

- Immunity. Aerobic exercise, explains *Staying Young*, "stimulates the activity of immune cells and makes your whole immune system work better." "You'll be setting up a strong line of defense against a variety of diseases," says Willix.

If all of these improvements to body systems don't increase your life expectancy, then it's hard to imagine what would.

WHAT ABOUT FREE RADICALS?

There's a catch to aerobics, says Bortz. "The accelerated traffic in oxygen does result in increased generation of potentially harmful free radicals, the same free radicals that are widely held to be responsible for the deteriorating changes associated with the aging process.

"So does exercise accelerate aging? No!"

Aerobic exercisers do generate more oxygen, but they also get rid of it faster than do other people. "The systems your body has developed to get rid of those free radicals are also increased by exercise," writes the University of Wales's Bellamy in *Ageing*. "There is no evidence that the tissues' antioxidant systems fail to take care of the increased production of free radicals."

Even if the body does fail to take care of excess free radicals, the *Age Erasers* books note, "any [free-radical] damage is minimal with normal exercise and offset by the added benefits that exercise provides."

Therefore, in the aerobic exercise versus free radicals fight, exercise wins.

HOW HARD SHOULD YOU WORK OUT?

Although experts have developed formulas involving target heart rates and rates of perceived exertion, a rough consensus advocates reaching and maintaining a steady pace about half to three-quarters of the most all-out, punishingly strenuous exertion that you can achieve. At this half- to three-fourths rate, you'll probably be sweating and breathing hard, but you won't be straining toward collapse and exhaustion.

This moderately hard workout has medical advantages. "Aerobic exercise at moderate intensity lowers blood pressure more than a high-intensity workout," Ford says. Deeb explains, "A study done by Arthur Leon, M.D., of the University of Minnesota, showed that men who burned on average only 285 calories per day during activities such as walking, gardening, or fishing derived as much heart benefit as those who burned twice as many calories doing [more] strenuous aerobic exercises."

Whatever the intensity of the workout, the important thing is to keep it continuous. Starting and stopping doesn't provide benefits. As Fries says, "Aerobic activity can't come in bursts; it must be sustained."

SPECIFIC AEROBIC EXERCISES

WALKING

How useful is walking in living long?

- "It is the exercise overwhelmingly preferred by people over 70. Most persons who reach their 100th birthday have literally walked most of the way," Georgakas says.

- In *Ageless Body, Timeless Mind,* Chopra notes that in Abkhazia (in the former Soviet Union), a region famous for the longevity of its residents, "it was customary for people to walk distances up to 20 miles a day."

- "Each additional mile a sedentary person walks or runs can lengthen his life by 21 minutes," says *Live Longer, Live Better.*

How does walking work these miracles?

- It consumes calories. Chopra notes, "Walking uses up between 290 and 430 calories per hour, depending on how fast you walk." Brisk walking "will burn off three pounds of weight each month, more than is lost in most weight reduction programs," says Georgakas.

- As a weight-bearing exercise, walking can build bone—Fries says that it can fight off osteoporosis—and increase muscle all over the body. As Barnard explains, "Your torso moves with every step, and your arms move actively from the shoulders. Your neck muscles work to keep your head in balance, toning themselves in the process."

- Walking also helps the heart, lungs, back, digestion, blood pressure, and other organs and systems.

To get these benefits, it's best to walk properly.

How to walk

"Roll from heel to toe," advises *Staying Young*. "Land first on your heel, flexing your foot just before you do, then roll forward across the ball of the foot and push off with the toes."

Keep your shoulders relaxed and your head erect and level but not ramrod stiff. Stand straight; don't bend forward. "As you step forward, the hip motion is forward, not side to side," *Live Longer, Live Better* adds.

Where you walk isn't all that important; some experts recommend using a track, others a scenic route. But no matter where you go, advises *Live Longer, Live Better*, occasionally change direction to avoid putting excess stress on any single side or part of the body.

Walk fast. "Walking by itself is not always an aerobic exercise," says Fries. "You need to push the pace quite a bit to break a sweat and get your heart rate up. Walking uphill or upstairs can quite quickly become aerobic." More precisely, Willix adds: "Walk about three or four miles per hour, or approximately 120 or 140 steps per minute."

If walking briskly is better than walking slowly, is even more strenuous activity better still? Not necessarily. Georgakas believes that walking is better than more strenuous exercises such as running in place or skipping rope. Walking, he explains, is less likely to cause stiffness, physical stress, or cramps.

"Don't forget about the importance of correct footwear," Fries cautions. *Live Longer, Live Better* says that the insole should give strong arch support and cushioning; the outsole should be durable, springy, and rubbery; the tongue should be padded; and the toe box should be roomy enough for you to wiggle your toes while standing. As *Staying Young* puts it, "You want about a half-inch between your big toe and the front end of the shoe."

Once you get used to walking, consider a slightly stronger workout: speeding the pace, walking up and down hills, swinging the arms, carrying weights, adding short jogs to your walks, or any combination of these options.

RUNNING

Running is one of the exercises that the experts prescribe most. As both a weight-bearing and an aerobic exercise, it can strengthen the body, relax the mind, wash out toxins such as LDL cholesterol, improve the functioning of the cardiovascular system, and, in all probability, increase longevity.

Running even has an advantage over walking—time. "Twenty minutes of running is approximately comparable to between 40 and 60 minutes of brisk walking," says *Live Longer, Live Better*.

But unlike walking, running is likely to bring injuries.

"Running . . . is longevously problematic, due to the stress it brings to the joints," explains Georgakas. According to *Live Longer*, the pounding of feet on the ground or track can cause injuries ranging from inflammation and muscle strains to sprains and stress fractures.

Fortunately, a runner can avoid injuries. Here are some popular methods.

- Get good shoes. "Buy running shoes that fit properly (your toes shouldn't be cramped), support your feet, and absorb shock," advises *Live Longer*.

- Run on a soft surface. "Hard surfaces, such as concrete, significantly intensify long-term wear-and-tear damage," says Georgakas. *Live Longer, Live Better* agrees: "Pick a forgiving running surface such as a cushioned synthetic indoor or outdoor track, a grassy field, or a dirt road."

- Don't sprint or race. "Speed events . . . may put severe pressure on the joints and organs," warns Georgakas. "Running very rapidly over a short course . . . is debilitating." He adds, "Rather than promoting the steady oxygen efficiency that is of benefit in daily life, racing is a severe test which swiftly draws extraordinary amounts of oxygen from the lungs. This sudden oxygen withdrawal is so enormous that the stress can trigger a heart attack."

- Don't run marathons. "Long-distance running may actually dampen your immune system," Mindell says. "[Long-distance] runners are more prone to colds, flu, and upper-respiratory ailments after participating in a marathon. Researchers suspect that overexertion may have a weakening effect on the body."

A note about running's little brother, jogging: "What most people refer to as jogging is actually running," Georgakas says. "True jogging involves a pace just a bit faster than walking. Its only advantage over walking is that it achieves the same cardiovascular benefits in a shorter space of time. Its danger is that jogging usually turns into running."

But if you take care to avoid injuries and other problems, running can be a very effective exercise for longevity.

SWIMMING

While not a weight-bearing exercise like walking or running—the water, not the exerciser, is bearing the body's weight—swimming has its own advantages.

- "Swimming is an ideal aerobic exercise," says *Live Longer, Live Better*. It can reduce stress, keep the body flexible, and aid the cardiovascular system. "A half-hour of swimming will give you a whole-body aerobic workout," says *Staying Young*.

- Swimming even outdoes dry aerobics in a few areas. It burns calories faster than hiking, cycling, or dancing, as well as such nonaerobic exercises as skiing, weight training, tennis, or house cleaning. Georgakas calls it "unbeatable for its overall toning by virtue of working every muscle in the body." It's especially good, says *Live Longer, Live Better*, at toning the muscles of the upper body.

- Another advantage: a low rate of injury. "Your joints will not be subjected to the strains that most other physical activities involve," Ryback says. After all, as *Live Longer, Live Better* says, swimming is a low-impact activity that does its job "without jarring bones or joints."

The best stroke for burning calories is the backstroke—although Georgakas notes, "Any stroke is prolongevous as long as the swimming is continuous."

To keep the swimming continuous, Willix says, "alternate between a work stroke (like the freestyle) and a rest stroke (like the sidestroke) so you will be able to swim for 30 consecutive minutes or more."

Drawbacks

For all of its advantages, swimming can create some problems.

- Watch out for the sun. Ryback warns, "If your aerobic activity is outdoor swimming, you're under the sun on a routine basis"—and too much sunlight can harm the skin. Ryback recommends water-resistant sunblock—or even better, waterproof sunblock—as skin protection. And *Live Longer, Live Better* advises, "Reapply sunscreen after swimming."

- Swimming can get deadly boring. "Doing laps in a pool or swimming back and forth across the same lake may become tedious as a daily enterprise," says Georgakas.

  To avoid this problem, try different strokes, use equipment such as kickboards, or alternate swimming with other exercises, such as walking. Janet Katz, City University of New York physical-education professor and a former Olympic swimmer, says, "You can walk or 'run' back and forth in the shallow end of a swimming pool or do a variety of water calisthenics, and get a great aerobic workout."

- Ryback warns, "You may lose weight a bit more slowly than in running because you'll tend to build more muscle [when] swimming." If this is one of swimming's drawbacks, it's one that most people would be happy to live with.

Overall, then, swimming is one of the best aerobic exercises.

CYCLING

Whether it's done on a track, cross-country, or on a stationary bike, cycling is good aerobic exercise.

Live Longer, Live Better explains, "Bicycling is a calorie-burning, heart-rate-raising activity that lets you cover far greater distances than walking or jogging and is gentler on your joints"—and it's "excellent for aerobic endurance and weight control."

Like swimming, "cycling may not result in nearly as much muscle destruction" as high-impact sports such as running, says Arnot. Unless you actually fall off your bike, you're unlikely to suffer injuries.

Arnot summarizes some of cycling's other advantages. "Training on a great bike rewards you with a dynamic cardiovascular system, springy powerful muscles, and the body of a much younger man. Exercise physiologists asked to pick just one piece of exercise equipment for a desert island most frequently select a bicycle. They know they can get strength, speed, endurance, agility, balance, and coordination training all on a single piece of equipment that is also a lot of fun."

How to ride

Willix advises, "When pedaling, keep your knees in close and your heels flat." To avoid spills, shocks, and injuries when going over bumps in the road, *Live Longer, Live Better* says, "Raise your buttocks off the seat . . . [and] keep your elbows slightly bent for better shock absorption."

Equipment is important. *Live Longer, Live Better* says, "A salesperson at a reputable bike shop can help you select one with the correct frame size (which is not adjustable) and set the seat and handlebars at the right height for you." *Live Longer* recommends that the bike's seat and handlebars be easy to adjust.

Specifically, Willix advises, "Adjust your seat so there is a 15- to 20-degree bend in your knee when the pedal is at six o'clock (the bottom of the stroke)."

For safety's sake, adds *Live Longer, Live Better*, "Take your bike in for a yearly tune-up, and check brakes, gears, and tires before every outing."

Almost as important as the bike is the helmet. "Always wear a helmet," advises *Live Longer, Live Better*. "It should have a sticker saying it meets or surpasses the standards of the American National Standards Institute or the Snell Memorial Foundation."

Cycling isn't perfect. The experts aren't in complete agreement as to how much it helps the upper body.

But no one disputes that it's an excellent source of aerobic exercise.

HIGH-IMPACT AND LOW-IMPACT AEROBICS

Live Longer, Live Better lists aerobics—the Lycra-leotard kind offered on videotapes and in health-club classes—among the best aerobic exercises. But watch out.

"High-impact aerobics such as those made popular in the early videotapes of Jane Fonda, exercises in which both feet leave the floor, should be avoided due to their jolting effect and joint stress," says Georgakas.

Low-impact aerobics are another story. They're "excellent for aerobic fitness and overall body toning," says *Live Longer, Live Better*. They also deliver less chance of injury.

Even with low-impact aerobics, Georgakas says, "Be wary of health club classes. The instructors are not medically trained, and most of the routines they favor involve movements that are antilongevous in their speed, stress, and intimacy." Georgakas adds that his warnings about instructors also apply to "most exercise tapes put out by movie stars and other celebrities."

To pick an instructor, in person or on tape, find out his or her certification. "Make sure the instructor is certified by one of the following: the American College of Sports Medicine, the American Council on Exercise, the Aerobics and Fitness Association of America, or the Cooper Institute for Aerobics Research," recommends *Live Longer, Live Better*.

OTHER AEROBIC EXERCISES

Among the other aerobic exercises most often mentioned by the experts are dancing, skating, cross-country skiing, rowing, and stair climbing. As long as you do them briskly, continuously, safely, and regularly, they should provide health benefits useful in living a long life.

STRENGTH BUILDING

Call it strength building, resistance training, progressive resistance, strength training, or building lean muscle mass—they're all the same, and the longevity experts recommend them.

BENEFITS OF STRENGTH

Strength building can improve cholesterol levels, self-esteem, blood circulation, mental ability, and recovery from disease. What's more:

- It aids weight control. *Live Longer, Live Better* notes that lifting weights burns more calories per minute than such fast-moving strenuous sports as gymnastics or volleyball. *Staying Young* says, "Resistance training . . . also speeds metabolism, which will cause your body to burn calories even while you're relaxing."

- It strengthens bones. "To increase bone density or to prevent bone thinning requires a combination of weight-bearing aerobic exercise *plus* strength-building exercises," Ford says. In fighting osteoporosis, "resistance training may be even more powerful [than aerobic exercise]," reports *Staying Young*.

- It can fight diabetes. Willix explains, "As the muscle mass in your body increases, your body needs less insulin to get sugar, or glucose, out of your blood and into your tissues, where it's required for energy. This means that your body is less likely to experience a shortage of insulin, making it less likely that you'll develop . . . diabetes."

Or as Georgakas puts it, "When weights are kept light and strength is built mainly through repetition, there are longevity benefits."

DISADVANTAGES AND DANGERS

Weight lifting is not aerobic, says *Live Longer, Live Better*. "Activities that . . . require exertion only in short bursts (such as weight lifting or football) are not considered aerobic and do not improve aerobic fitness."

Another danger: "Resistance training may cause surges in blood pressure," the *Age Erasers* books say. A cause of those surges, says *Live Longer, Live Better*, is holding your breath, which "can cause your blood pressure to rise dangerously. Instead, exhale as you lift the weight and inhale as you bring the weight down."

Unusually heavy weights can be dangerous, too. "Professional muscle men do not enjoy long life spans," says Georgakas. "To lift extraordinarily heavy weights, the lifter must have layers and layers of fat to support the overdeveloped muscles. The jerking motions involved in the actual lifting place sudden and possibly traumatic demands upon the heart."

But if you train carefully and combine weights with aerobic exercise, weight lifting can safely provide longevity benefits.

WORKOUT ADVICE

- Check with your doctor. Says *Staying Young*, "Talk to your doctor or physical therapist before starting a weight-training program. This advice is particularly important if your doctor has said you may be at risk for osteoporosis or other health conditions." Among those other conditions are high blood pressure, heart disease, or any other serious medical problem.

- Warm up. If you get the doctor's okay, start your workout by warming up. Many experts recommend stretching the muscles that you plan to strengthen. Stretch gently, and vary the different types of stretches. This warm-up should take about five minutes.

- Know your form. "Technique is as important as weight," says Willix. Knowing how to do the exercises will give you the maximum benefits of the exercise and keep injuries away. As Ryback points out, "Doing the wrong thing in the beginning (starting with weights that are too heavy, performing too many reps, or following the wrong sequence or combination of exercises) can really put a dent in your workout. Seek a trainer's advice."

- Start out easy. Use light weights at first. As Bortz says, "Don't push it, but keep it up."

  Most experts recommend using weights that you can lift over and over again, from eight to twenty times, with the average being about twelve. Such a group of repetitions is called a set.

  If you're up to doing more than one set, says Live Longer, Live Better, "Let your muscles recover between sets." "The time you spend resting between individual sets allows your muscle enzymes to replenish and permits you to lift a weight again and again without damage," Willix explains. The rest period should last from 30 seconds to 3 minutes, depending on how soon you feel ready to continue the workout.

- Go big. "Work the large muscle groups (legs, back, chest, arms) first," says *Live Longer, Live Better.* Why? *Staying Young* explains that working the big ones first "will increase circulation, which will improve your endurance and allow you to exercise longer before tiring."

- Do the whole body. "Include all muscles in your total workout plan," says *Live Longer.* "Also, equally work the muscles in opposing pairs—hamstrings on the back of the thigh and quadriceps on the front of the thigh, for example."

  One way to make sure that you're using all your muscles, says Bortz, is to "use standing, sitting, and lying as starting postures for the exercises, because each one provides a chance to use different muscle groups." Varying the exercises can also help to prevent over-straining any single muscle group.

- Cool down. After the workout, do a cool-down that's roughly similar to the warm-up, the experts say. Willix on cool-downs: "I recommend an easy stretching session and some easy jogging or walking for about five minutes following your weight-training exercise. This will help you to avoid strain and injury."

- Rest. "Never work the same muscles on consecutive days; muscles need 24 hours to recover," advises *Live Longer, Live Better.*

   Willix agrees, prescribing a workout routine in which "the chest, shoulders, and triceps would be exercised two days (Monday and Thursday, for example), and the legs, back, and biceps would be exercised two of the other days (Tuesday and Friday, for example)."

- Keep it up. Make sure that the repetitions challenge you enough to continue delivering longevity benefits.

"How do you know when an exercise is not giving you the benefits you want?" Willix asks—and answers, "As soon as the exercise becomes too easy. In other words, as soon as you have strengthened a muscle or a group of muscles enough that you are able to do sets of ten or twelve repetitions without resting for more than a few seconds between each set—it's time to make the exercise more difficult."

How to make it more difficult? "Either increase the number of repetitions or the amount of weight (but not both at once)," recommends *Live Longer, Live Better.* If you do the latter, then "increase the amount of weight you use gradually," Bortz cautions. "Never overextend."

After all, getting injured is no way to increase longevity.

A last word

Staying Young adds one final (and probably welcome) bit of advice on strength exercises: "Stop if you're in pain. . . . A mild burning sensation is normal with resistance efforts, but any acute or stabbing pain is a warning that you are straining too hard or performing the maneuver incorrectly."

CLUBS, GYMS, TRAINERS, AND PARTNERS

Strength training isn't easy or stimulating to do alone. Many authorities recommend getting someone to help.

Health clubs and gyms

To learn how to use weights properly, go to a gym or health club. To pick a good club, follow a few basic criteria.

The club should be near your home or office so that you'll be able to use it conveniently and often. It should be clean and have the equipment—free weights or machines—that you prefer to use. Visit the club at the times when you'll want to use it, and make sure that it's not so crowded at those times that you'll have to wait a long time for equipment or instruction.

Make sure that the instruction suits you. Sit in on classes, talk to the trainers, and see if the trainers are willing to listen and eager to help.

Trainers

Know what you're getting.

"There are many people out there claiming to be qualified exercise trainers but who have few qualifications," Mindell says. *Live Longer, Live Better* advises, "Trainers should have a background in exercise physiology, kinesiology, or physical education."

When seeking a strength trainer, look for one with the proper accreditation. Many experts praise the American College of Sports Medicine as trustworthy when it comes to certifying trainers. Other organizations with good reputations include the American Council on Exercise, the Cooper Institute for Aerobics Research, the Aerobics and Fitness Association of America, and the National Strength and Conditioning Association.

Finally, says Aronne, "Don't work with instructors who bully or intimidate you. Remember, exercise should be fun!"

Partners

Whether you work out at a health club or at home, get a partner.

This advice crops up in discussions of almost all exercise, but it's especially common in strength training. "It's more fun to have company, and you're less likely to slack off if another person is counting on you," says Mindell.

Into the future

Now that you're ready to begin, it's on to the details:

- the strength exercises you should perform;

- the distinctions among them;

- and how you should perform them.

SPECIFIC STRENGTH EXERCISES

"There are many different exercises for each muscle group," the *Age Erasers* books say. Exercise physiologist Alan Mikesky says, "If you don't like an exercise, don't stay with it. Find one you like."

There are obviously more exercises than the few that are listed here. These are simply ones that the longevity literature recommends often. Since this isn't a workout book, anyone with interest in these or other strength exercises should consult a trainer.

CALISTHENICS

You may groan at the thought of calisthenics—they probably remind you of junior-high phys ed—but they have their benefits. Willix calls calisthenics "one of the oldest and easiest forms of exercise." Ford adds, "You can begin a strength-building program without weights or machines by using calisthenics alone. This is a great way to get started."

How do calisthenics build strength without heavy lifting? "Calisthenics, such as chin-ups, push-ups, and sit-ups, utilize your own body weight as the resistance force," explain the *Age Erasers* books.

A few well-known and often-recommended calisthenics:

Sit-ups

Lie down on your back with your arms folded on your chest or your hands behind your head. Gently raise your shoulders toward your knees and slowly lower them back down.

The abdominal muscles are the target of this exercise. If other parts of the body are feeling more strain than the gut, either you're doing the exercise improperly or you have a physical problem that may require medical attention.

Chin-ups

Grab a horizontal bar and hang from it. Pull yourself up until your chin clears the bar. Lower yourself back down to where you started.

Arnot says that the chin-up strengthens the back. He adds, "Plan on doing fifty chin-ups at a sitting. You may eke out only three or four per set, but still try to force your way through to a total of fifty."

Push-ups

Lie face down, elbows bent, hands beside your shoulders, legs extended. Slowly push your body up, keeping it in a rigid line, until your weight rests only on your arms and your toes or on your arms and the balls of your feet. Bend the elbows, slowly lowering yourself until you're back down to the floor.

When you do this exercise, says Willix, "you strengthen major muscles in your arms, chest, shoulders, and back."

A softer version of this exercise allows you to raise your body so that your knees as well as your toes and arms touch the floor. In either case, your back should remain straight.

STRENGTH TRAINING WITH EQUIPMENT

"There are two basic kinds of weight-training equipment: free weights (barbells and dumbbells) and weight machines," says *Live Longer, Live Better*.

Willix defines barbells as long bars with weights at each end and dumbbells as weight-carrying bars short enough to be grasped by one hand.

Weight machines, he says, include "the standard weight/stack pulley arrangement, with which you increase or decrease resistance by adding or removing weights that are then pulled or pushed using bars and a system of pulleys; rubber cable systems, which use a variety of adjusting devices to increase or decrease resistance; [and] shock absorber systems, which also use various devices to adjust resistance."

Which is better? Both have advantages and disadvantages. For the beginner, it's probably better to try both under the eye of a qualified trainer and see which one you like better.

FREE-WEIGHT EXERCISES

There are many more free-weight exercises than this volume can fit, but here are some of the better known ones:

Curls

Curls, such as the arm curl, are among the most common exercises with free weights. Performed sitting or standing while holding weights in one or both hands, the arm curl is done by curling the weight up toward the chest and down toward the thighs.

There are several types of arm curls, as well as curls to strengthen other parts of the body.

Presses

Presses are another kind of popular free-weight strengthener. Two examples:

The bench press exercises the chest. Lie on the floor or on a bench, lift the weights from the chest until the elbows are only slightly bent, and back down to the chest.

The overhead press strengthens the upper part of the body, particularly the arms. Start with your hands holding the weights at about shoulder level, with elbows bent; then extend the arms (and weights) upward; and bring them down again.

Lateral raise

This shoulder strengthener is another frequently used free-weight exercise. "This one can be performed with dumbbells or a machine," Arnot says.

Starting with the arms down and a weight in each hand, slowly—without bending the elbows—raise the arms. The arms should be extended out to the sides, not very far forward or back. Stop when the hands and weights reach shoulder level. Then lower the weights slowly back to the starting position.

RESISTANCE MACHINE EXERCISES

Abdominal crunch, bent-forward cable crossover, decline seated cable row, triceps press-down—the range of exercises that can be performed on resistance machines is as complex as the machines themselves. Here are a popular few:

Rowing machine exercises

Ford notes that using a rowing machine at a moderate pace is good not just for strength but also for aerobic power, because it burns 325 calories per hour—almost as many as in brisk walking. And *Live Longer, Live Better* calls rowing "excellent for upper-body and leg strength and endurance." A variety of different exercises are available on rowing machines.

Lat pull-downs

Arnot recommends lat pull-downs, especially if you're just starting to train for the first time. Lat pull-downs exercise the back muscles, known as the *latissimus dorsi*.

On a lat machine, the exerciser sits while holding a horizontal bar that hangs by a cord above his head. The exerciser should use a palms-forward overhand grip on the bar. The exerciser slowly pulls the bar down until it touches his upper chest and then slowly lets the bar up again. The amount of resistance that the exerciser gets depends on the amount of weight that he sets in the machine.

Leg curl

This exercise—which, naturally, strengthens the legs—involves a bench with an adjustable stack of weight plates at one end and a roller pad (it looks like the business end of a paint roller) at the other, and a cord connecting the two. The exerciser lies down on the bench with his head facing the weight plates and his feet facing the roller pad.

The exerciser slips his heels under the roller pad. He raises the roller pad by lifting both feet until his soles are straight up and his leg, bent at the knee, forms a 90-degree angle. (The weight connected by the cord to the roller pad determines the amount of resistance that the exerciser must overcome.) Then the exerciser slowly lowers his feet to the starting position.

STRETCHING AND FLEXIBILITY

In themselves, stretching and flexibility don't extend life.

But they can influence the things that do. Stretching can help to reduce tension, decrease pain, increase strength, lower the chance of being injured (and repair injuries that already exist), and make it easier at any age to do the aerobic exercises and strength builders that help the body to live longer.

HOW TO STRETCH

- Get instruction. "Take a stretch and tone class at a local health club or Y," Mindell advises. "Even if you just attend one stretch class weekly, you can do the exercises at home on your own."

- Warm up. The experts recommend a few minutes of walking or jogging. Deeb adds, "Go slowly. Never try to rush your muscles into a warm-up! Not only will a hurried warm-up risk injury, but you will also lose much of the benefit to your muscles."

- Stretch slowly. A slow stretch is the likeliest way to get the most effect with the least chance of injury.

- Hold it. When you do a stretch, don't unstretch right away. Hold the stretch. The experts disagree as to exactly how long you should hold it; their recommendations range from three seconds to two minutes. For a beginner, it's probably good to hold the stretch for only a few seconds.

- Don't bounce. "[Bouncing] is a sure way to be injured," says Bortz.

- Be gentle. "Don't force muscles to stretch; gently allow them to move into the tight zone, test the resistance, and relax. Each day, you can slightly increase the stretching of that tight zone," advises *Staying Young*.

- If it hurts, stop. "The increased activity of a new fitness program may tighten muscles at first," concedes Deeb. "A whimper of protest [from the body] may mean that your body is simply unaccustomed to a new or increased movement which it really should make." But anything worse than a whimper may indicate that you're doing something wrong.

Fortunately, as Bortz points out, "The more you stretch, the easier it becomes."

SOME SPECIFIC STRETCHES

The hamstring stretch (a thigh stretcher)

Lie flat on your back. Bend a leg and pull it toward your chest. Then straighten the leg out as much as you can, so that it is aiming straight up (or as close to straight up as you can get). Repeat the process with the other leg.

The angry cat stretch (also called the cat and dog stretch)
The angry cat stretch makes your trunk more flexible. Get on your hands and knees with your back level and parallel to the floor. Arch your back like an angry cat, lowering your head and sucking in your stomach muscles. Hold that pose for a few seconds. Then return to the starting position.

The quadriceps stretch
This one stretches the leg. Stand next to a chair or wall. With your left hand on the chair or wall for balance, bend your right leg, bringing your foot up behind you. With your right hand, grasp the right ankle and pull it up (gently!) toward your buttocks. Let the leg down and repeat the process with the left leg and hand.

YOGA

Although it involves stretching and flexibility, yoga—which means "union"—does much more than that.

"Yoga brings renewed youth," writes Ryback in *Look 10 Years Younger, Live 10 Years Longer*. More precisely, yoga can lower blood pressure, reduce stress, build strength, and relieve pain. "It has become an important part of post-heart-attack rehabilitation in many hospitals," says Ford.

What is yoga?
Willix says, "Yoga is—at its simplest—a system for achieving mind–body harmony in which you assume postures or 'asanas' and practice breathing that enables you to relax and control your body."

Ford, who describes yoga as "[a] combination of breathing, stretching, and balancing," explains, "Yoga functions on a holistic level which limbers up the body while it also calms the mind."

Learning how

"Yoga requires instruction from a knowledgeable teacher," advises *Live Longer, Live Better*, and many other experts agree.

Based on advice from Alice Christensen of the American Yoga Association, the *Age Erasers* books suggest "looking for a teacher who practices yoga every day and sees his own yoga teacher on a regular basis. Ask the teacher for references. Take a trial class before you invest long-term time or money. And if you have specific problems, like a bad back or arthritis, make sure you find a teacher who will individualize instruction for you."

Although classes are the preferred way to go, Ford says, "You can learn the postures from a book or videotape." The *Age Erasers* books report that the American Yoga Association has a correspondence course; its address is 513 South Orange Avenue, Sarasota, Florida 34236.

Be careful with yoga

"Going too far will injure you," Christensen warns.

"Unless performed correctly, some stretches could conceivably pop a muscle or cause a minor injury," Ford says. "Stop immediately if pain occurs [during a stretch] and avoid that stretch until fully recovered."

The *Age Erasers* books add, "Stretch slowly and evenly. Don't bounce. And push only as far as your body lets you."

Also, remember that yoga is not aerobic and can't take the place of aerobic exercise.

BEYOND THE BOUNDARIES

Some activities aren't exactly aerobic or strength-building or promoters of flexibility. But they're good exercises with strong records of increasing longevity.

T'AI CHI

The experts love t'ai chi. Willix recommends it "if you cannot perform aerobic activity because of some physical condition." Georgakas describes it as "high on the prolongevity scale."

T'ai chi (also known by its full name, t'ai chi ch'uan) is a Chinese system of exercising in slow, rhythmic movements. "T'ai chi adepts employ flowing contemplative poses to enhance suppleness, to cultivate a balance of two inner forces called yin and yang, and to achieve serenity and detachment," explains *Search for Immortality*.

T'ai chi can build strength and flexibility, and lower some stresses. It is unlikely to cause injuries. And it's usually inexpensive.

Many health clubs offer t'ai chi instruction. Ask the instructor if you can observe or participate in a class, and see how you like it.

NONEXERCISE EXERCISES

Maybe you hate exercise. You're in good company. A lot of people do—even people who are perfect examples of longevity. Chopra, as a matter of fact, mentions a study of centenarians that found "a marked absence of pursuing organized exercise."

So what do they do instead? "As long as you perform regular minimal activity—the equivalent of walking half an hour a day—you are gaining most of the longevity benefits conferred by exercise," Chopra says.

Some examples:

Breathing

Believe it or not, breathing can be exercise. Proper breathing can aid sleep and improve lung capacity.

But its greatest power is as a stress reliever. *Staying Young* explains, "It works its magic by infusing the blood with extra oxygen and causing the body to release endorphins, the natural tranquilizing hormones." In fact, Dr. Dean Ornish of the Preventive Medicine Research Institute, says, "Deep breathing is one of the simplest yet most effective stress-management techniques there is."

How should you breathe? There are several methods, some to be done while seated, some while standing, and still others while lying down. Most of them share this advice:

- Go slow. Whether inhaling or exhaling, do it gently and easily and without rushing.

- Breathe deeply. *Live Longer* speaks for many experts when it says, "[Use] your diaphragm, the dome-shaped muscle below the lungs that contracts to expand [the lungs] to their full capacity."

- Feel the breath enter and exit your body. "Pay attention to the gentle rising and falling of your abdomen, the movement of your ribs, or the sensation of the breath moving through your nostrils," advise the *Age Erasers* books.

- Think good thoughts. "Recapture the feeling of being happy, vibrant, and carefree," Chopra says. The *Age Erasers* books recommend, "As you breathe in, think to yourself, 'Cool clear mind.' Then, as you blow out, think, 'Calm, relaxed body.'" Aronne suggests, "As you exhale, visualize yourself letting go of pent-up stress."

- Repeat this procedure for at least five minutes.

Finding exercise in everyday activities

If you keep your eyes open to opportunity, you can get life-lengthening exercise without ever seeing the inside of a gym. DiGiovanna says, "Substituting muscle power for convenience can achieve real gains."

For example:

- Walk, don't drive. Some experts suggest leaving the car at home. Shopping or going to work by foot or bicycle, if possible, is good exercise. And if you must drive, DiGiovanna says, "Parking farther from stores [or the office] and walking to reach them . . . can significantly increase a person's amount of exercise."

- Take stairs instead of elevators or escalators. Ford notes that vigorous stair climbing burns 675 calories per hour—more than in cross-country skiing or using a rowing machine.

- Garden. Chopra lists gardening as one of the regular physical activities (along with active sports and long walks) characteristic of people who have lived a long time. Georgakas writes, "Gardening, with its multiple demands on the body, scores extremely well on the longevity scale."

  He adds, "When briskly done, movements like hoeing, digging, and raking for an hour at a time are equivalent or superior to jogging. Bending to pull weeds, staking up plants, tugging at sacks of manure, and other strenuous chores tote up numerous pluses for the muscular-skeletal system."

  Even something as simple as lawn mowing is surprisingly good exercise. Live Longer, Live Better notes that it burns more calories per minute than tennis, cycling, weight lifting, gymnastics, or golf, and more than twice as much as volleyball.

  But there is a danger in gardening. Mindell notes that lawn and garden chemicals that promote plant growth "can disrupt normal biological processes in humans."

  Fortunately, Mindell goes on to say, "there are many natural toxin-free lawn and garden products on the market that can do the job just as well. Check your local plant nursery, natural food store, or botanical gardens for information on environmentally friendly gardening techniques."

SPORTS

Football, baseball, basketball, hockey, tennis, golf, volleyball—they're fun, exciting, and popular, but they're not the best exercises for aerobics, strength building, or flexibility. They often have a herky-jerky, start-and-stop rhythm that isn't as beneficial as steadily walking, stretching, or lifting weights.

Moreover, the high risk of injury in some sports—particularly football and hockey—makes them less than conducive to longevity.

If you like sports, play them. They're unquestionably better than no exercise at all. Besides, you're more likely to participate in sports than in activities that you don't enjoy.

But give walking, rowing, calisthenics, swimming, the hamstring stretch, yoga, or t'ai chi a try. They're better for longevity, and you might enjoy them just as much as golf or hockey.

PART FOUR:
WAYS OF LIVING

DIET, EXERCISE, AND STRESS REDUCTION AREN'T THE ONLY MEANS TO long life. A whole system of activities and ways of living can lengthen—or shorten—the years.

TRAINING THE MIND

OPTIMISM

As noted in the section of this book on the longevity profile, long-lived people are optimistic, active, and resilient. If that description doesn't cover you, take heart. There are clear, simple ways to get a long-living personality.

- Think happily. "Concentrate on an accomplishment or an experience, however minor, that has given you pleasure," advises *Staying Young*. *The Age Erasers* books add, "Take credit [for your achievements]." If you're facing trouble, *Staying Young* suggests telling yourself, "I know what to do to make progress," "What I don't know I can learn," and other affirmations.

- Prefer specific explanations to general ones. Asks *Staying Young*, "If you flub a presentation at work, is it because you're terrible at public speaking or because you didn't prepare as well as usual? The first reason is pervasive and pessimistic; the second specific and optimistic." The *Age Erasers* books add, "Don't confuse belief with fact"—that is, don't call yourself a loser if you're just having some bad times.

- Stop the bad thoughts. If your view of a situation is pessimistic, "distract yourself," *Staying Young* says. "Then, while the negative thought is interrupted, replace it with another thought"—a more optimistic one.

- Create your own goals. "Self-esteem can come from self-generated goals and accomplishments as opposed to externally awarded grades and promotions," David Ryback, Ph.D., says in *Look Ten Years Younger, Live Ten Years Longer.*

- Spend satisfying time with others. *The Age Erasers* books advise helping people in need and seeking out people with a positive attitude. If you run into a conflict with others, *Staying Young* recommends, "Phrase disagreements in ways that focus on how [you] feel, rather than accusing or blaming the other person."

- Envision better times. "Researchers at Washington State University in Pullman found that visualization [of positive images and outcomes] significantly lowered apprehension," reports *Staying Young.*

These methods offer a bonus to simply extending life. They make the years not just longer but, in all probability, happier.

RELAXATION AND STRESS REDUCTION

Relaxation and stress reduction can control pain, improve cholesterol levels, balance hormones, and improve circulation, all of which can help to lead to longer life.

- In *Healthy at 100,* heart surgeon Robert Willix reports on "a large-scale study of 2,000 older health-insurance customers. . . . Those who followed a daily routine of relaxation exercises had 87 percent fewer instances of heart disease than normal for their age group, 55 percent fewer cancerous tumors, and 87 percent fewer nervous disorders."

- "[A] study conducted jointly by Maharishi International University, Harvard University, and the University of Maryland found that seniors who meditated for three months experienced dramatic improvements in their psychological well-being, compared to their nonmeditative peers," writes author Katherine Greider in the November–December 1996 issue of *Psychology Today*.

The most frequently suggested form of stress reduction is exercise, which Willix calls "the ultimate stress management technique."

Besides exercise, here are several other ways to reduce stress:

MEDITATION

Most experts recommend meditating for 15 to 30 uninterrupted minutes every day. Meditation can improve the heart and blood pressure and in general relieve stress and its life-shortening effects.

Three of the best-known kinds of meditation are "relaxation response" meditation, progressive relaxation, and transcendental meditation.

Relaxation response meditation

Harvard Medical School's Herbert Benson, an expert on meditation, has created a way to reach what he calls the "relaxation response"—the condition of being physically relaxed.

To trigger the relaxation response, find a quiet environment. Settle into a comfortable position (sitting, for instance) that decreases muscle tension. Breathe rhythmically and deeply. Sink into a passive attitude. Focus on a word or phrase unrelated to the situation around you. Repeat it silently to move the mind away from the external world. Eventually, your body should respond by relaxing—hence the relaxation response.

Repeating a word or phrase is not the only way to achieve the relaxation response. "Prayer can be an effective way to evoke the stress-relieving relaxation response," says *Staying Young*. The book quotes Benson: "Eighty percent of my patients chose a word or prayer arising from their faith." It seems to work. As Georgakas writes in *The Methuselah Factors*, "Not a few longevous people use prayer to buffer stress."

Whatever method you choose, Benson says, "The key is to find one method you're comfortable with and stick with it."

Progressive relaxation

"This simple exercise . . . involves focusing on each part of the body individually and isolating tense spots," explains *Live Longer, Live Better*. "By alternately tightening each set of muscles, then loosening them, you can gradually relax your entire body from head to toe."

The *Age Erasers* books add, "It should take about 10 minutes to complete the entire sequence [of the body's muscles]. Try to do these exercises twice a day."

A tight schedule isn't necessary, though. "When you become skillful [in progressive relaxation], you can use this technique to produce relaxation quickly any time you need to and in almost any environment," advises the *Complete Guide to Symptoms, Illness & Surgery for People Over 50*.

Transcendental meditation

It sounds gooey and unscientific, but transcendental meditation can be good for longevity. *Search for Immortality* explains, "A 1989 report on a study by five Harvard scholars actually concluded that transcendental meditation, as taught by the Maharishi Mahesh Yogi, could 'literally extend human life.'" And in a UCLA study, people who had been using TM for less than five years were five years younger in biological age than in chronological age. Moreover, the meditators had half the cancer rate of nonmeditators and 80 percent less heart disease.

So what is transcendental meditation? Chopra writes in *Ageless Body, Timeless Mind*, "TM is based on the silent meditation of a specific Sanskrit word, or mantra, whose sound vibrations gradually lead the mind out of its normal thinking process and into the silence that underlies thought." It is similar to relaxation response meditation, and provides similar results.

"TM is not something that you can learn to do by reading a book," Willix warns. Chopra agrees: "To learn it properly, one should receive personal instruction from a trained TM teacher."

OTHER WAYS TO HANDLE STRESS

Know thyself

Your body, says *Live Longer*, "can tell you when you're fielding too much stress." Chopra advises, "When choosing a certain behavior, ask your body, 'How do you feel about this?' If your body sends a signal of physical or emotional distress, watch out." Common signals include headache, backache, muscle tension, stomach trouble, and lack of sleep.

Get your priorities straight

Part of knowing yourself—and avoiding stress—is to "have a clear understanding of what's really important to you," Willix says. "Start by asking what your real goals are for yourself, your family, and your career," advises *Live Longer, Live Better*. Health journalist Sue Browder has reported a finding of Dr. Robert Butler from New York's Mount Sinai School of Medicine: "People who live the longest have strong interests and goals."

And once you set your goals . . .

Make a schedule

Keep a daily list of things to do. First on the list should be tasks that help you reach your most important goals. If you have too many tasks to complete, *Live Longer* advises, "Let go of activities . . . that don't contribute to your goals."

Make plenty of time for the activities that do. "By allotting yourself enough time to accomplish a task, you cut back on anxiety," the *Age Erasers* books advise.

One thing to make time for is, surprisingly, anxiety itself. "If you're stressed by compulsive worrying, set aside a half-hour the same time each day to focus on your worries," Ryback recommends.

Live Longer, Live Better explains, "Psychologist Roland Nathan believes that having a formal worrying time cuts down on the amount of worrying you do." Says Ryback, "If you're inclined to worry [at] any other time, just relegate your worries to your designated 'worry time' and get back to focusing on what you're doing."

Back, that is, to your goals and schedule.

Don't start

"'Avoid stress-inducing situations," says DiGiovanna in *Human Aging*. A good way to do this is to say no.

A friend asks you to help paint his house. You feel tightness in your gut or pain in your shoulder. You realize that as much as you might want to help your friend, you have more important goals and priorities for that particular weekend. If that's the case, it may be a good idea to beg off rather than accept the stress of letting a lower-priority task (painting *his* house) crowd out your more important goals.

But if you do get into stressful situations . . .

Get rid of the stressor

If possible, change or eliminate the conditions that are causing the stress. If doing so is especially difficult, Ryback suggests, "Solicit the support of the most capable professionals available to you—doctors, lawyers, financial experts. Give in to their expertise."

Eat right

Food can calm you. "Carbohydrates . . . trigger the release of hormones that will relax you," say the *Age Erasers* books. "So if you want to unwind at night, eat a plate of spaghetti, baked beans, or other complex carbohydrates for dinner."

Prepare the foods with garlic. Gilles Fillion of France's Pasteur Institute says, "Garlic affects the release of serotonin—a ubiquitous brain chemical involved in regulating a wide spectrum of moods and behavior, including anxiety . . . [and] stress."

Water matters, too, say the *Age Erasers* books. "Keep a plastic bottle of water at your desk and drink often. When you are under stress, you sweat more, and then of course, there's your dry mouth. You'll feel better if you hydrate your high anxiety."

On the other hand, avoid protein. Robert Eliot, M.D., says, "Protein seems to raise energy levels and keep you alert. . . . So if you have a hamburger late at night, you'll probably be rehashing yesterday's sales meeting until dawn."

Sleep right

"If you get less sleep than you need, you might wake feeling tense," say the *Age Erasers* books. A later section of this book will cover how much is enough.

Reach out

Friends are good for you. "It's important to feel accepted and appreciated by at least one social group," says Ryback. "Having a close supportive network reduces stress and promotes cardiovascular health."

The closer the network, the better. Intimate relationships are the best of all. "Psychologists tell us that intimacy is not only an immediate stress reducer, it also provides the kind of loving, nonjudgmental support that helps us develop confidence to deal with whatever life sends our way," *Staying Young* explains.

The sections of this book on marriage and family will give more detail on intimate relationships.

Let it out

"Express your anger," advises *Live Longer, Live Better*. "Cry if you feel like it." Do whatever it takes (short of a full-scale destructive blowup) to purge your stressful feelings.

Age Erasers for Men notes that you don't even have to take aim at the stressor itself. "You can blow off your emotions at a ball game and get some of the tension out of your system."

One of the best ways to let it out is through writing. "If you write about your problems, you can help relieve stress, improve your immunity, make fewer visits to the doctor, and have a more optimistic view of life," says James Pennebaker, Ph.D., professor of psychology at Southern Methodist University.

Different experts recommend different kinds of writing—diary entries, letters to friends, and so on. But they all agree that you should pour out your deepest emotions, insights, and stresses in as much detail as you can. It's a likely way to purge them.

Distract yourself

Get your mind as far from the stressors as you can.

- "Hobbies and other diversions can . . . provide relief [from stress]," DiGiovanna says. "Taking breaks or vacations from [stress-inducing] situations helps."

- Even a brief stroll may help. *Staying Young* says, "Walking helps dissipate harmful stress chemicals—instantly."

- Another method is music. "Scientific studies show that music played for patients before, during, or after surgery seems to reduce anxiety, lessen pain, and speed recovery," reports *Staying Young*.

- Or you can get wet. "Take a warm bath, and let stress go down the drain," says *Staying Young*. "Warm baths work by relaxing the muscles but also perhaps by slightly heating the brain, which can be calming."

  Staying Young notes, "Water between 100° and 102°F (that's comfortably warm to the touch) is best. Soak for . . . 15 minutes." But don't overdo it, advise the *Age Erasers* books: "Longer soaks in warmer water can actually lower your blood pressure too much."

Imagine

Visualizing scenes of nature in tranquillity is often effective in soothing yourself. The *Age Erasers* books suggest thinking of yourself on a warm beach or on a verdant mountain. *Staying Young* reports, "One study revealed that hospital patients whose rooms looked out on an area of trees recovered faster than those whose view was of a brick wall."

Besides visualizing nature, other ways to relax include the following:

- Conjure up memories of a happy carefree childhood.

- Think of a favorite painting or a piece of music.

- Ryback says, "Let your mind wander into your most delectable fantasy." If something soothes you, use it.

- Or you can even imagine catastrophe. "Imagine the worst possible outcome [of whatever situation is stressing you] and the consequences of that," advises Ryback. "In most cases by far, the outcome is not so severe, but by considering the worst, you can more easily deal with the rest."

Each person reacts differently. So choose among those options that suit you, and imagine whatever scene reduces your own stresses.

Laugh

It's hard to be stressful when you're in full-tilt guffaw.

"Humor is a proven stress reducer," say the *Age Erasers* books. "Laughter triggers the release of endorphins, chemicals in the brain that produce feelings of euphoria. It also suppresses the production of cortisol, a hormone released when you're under stress that indirectly raises blood pressure."

Laughter can relax muscles and reduce the perception of pain. The *Age Erasers* books explain, "Laughter can spur your immune system, increasing activity of lymphocytes and other 'killer cells' (antibodies) and possibly raising levels of disease-fighting immunoglobulin A in your bloodstream, according to Kathleen Dillon, Ph.D., a psychologist and professor at Western New England College in Springfield, Massachusetts."

Laughter being a spontaneous thing, how can you simply laugh on cue, especially when stressful times aren't funny? A common solution is to keep at hand anything that makes you laugh: cartoons, anecdotes, even a kid's windup toy.

Change your mind

"You are not stressed by *him* or by *that thing* or by *those events*. You are stressed by *your reactions to them*," says Willix.

And reactions you can change. Among the ways:

- Shift your viewpoint to make the stressor less serious.

Live Longer, Live Better says, "If you are terrified of public speaking, for example, try imagining the audience all naked. You may laugh, but once you have changed how you see that audience, it becomes less fearsome."

"You've suddenly lost your job," says Willix. "View the loss . . . not as a financial disaster but as an opportunity to find a better job and to grow and possibly make more money."

- Focus on process, not results. Chopra explains, "Stress always arises if you concentrate on how something *has* to turn out."

  To avoid this problem, says Chopra, "I remind myself that I don't need to know where I'm going to enjoy the road I'm on." Another method: "Keep in mind that there may be more than one solution to any dilemma," says *Live Longer, Live Better.*

- Finally, as Ryback says, "Realize the ultimate rule of overwhelming problems: This too shall pass!"

Seek therapy

If you try the above methods but stress continues to torture you, get professional help.

Many a stressed person has thought that getting help brands him a failure. But *Live Longer, Live Better* says, "Seeking assistance from a certified social worker, psychologist, or psychiatrist is not a sign of weakness or ineptitude. Instead, it suggests that you are willing and able to get the help you need."

How can you find a good counselor? *Live Longer* says, "Ask your friends or your doctors for recommendations, and don't be afraid to interview several therapists before settling on one."

What doesn't work

Don't use stimulants, relaxants, depressants, or other substances that monkey with the mind, emotions, and body. "If," Barnard writes in *Eat Right, Live Longer*, "we dose ourselves with increasing amounts of coffee or alcohol . . . we lose more control and become victims, not only of the original stresses, but [also] of our Band-Aid response to them."

Alcohol is of special concern. The *Age Erasers* books explain that it can disrupt sleep patterns and cause a stress-inducing feeling of being tired while wide awake.

Nor do seemingly healthier alternatives work. "Taking vitamin supplements," says *Live Longer, Live Better*, "is considered ineffective [as a stress fighter]. Although your body may need more vitamins and minerals during periods of physical stress (after surgery, for instance), mental stress does not appear to be relieved by vitamin formulas."

Finally, don't expect to get rid of all stress. As Willix points out, "There's no such thing as a stress-free life."

CONTROL OF YOUR LIFE

IF YOU FEEL IN CONTROL OF YOUR LIFE, YOU'LL FEEL LESS ANXIETY AND more ease—and you'll probably live longer.

- "When 1,200 centenarians were surveyed to find out their secret to longevity, 90 percent of the group identified the role of order in their lives," reports Bortz.

- University of Michigan aging researcher David Guttman says, "Active mastery . . . is the ego state most clearly associated with longevity." Active mastery, says Chopra, "means having autonomy over one's life and circumstances."

- In 1973, the University of Chicago's Dr. Bernice Neugarten presented a study of the kind of person who can live healthily to age 85 and older. Neugarten noted that this type of person feels a sense of achievement and that he's reached his most important goals.

HOW TO GET CONTROL

The experts recommend a variety of ways to control your life.

- Make plans. If you plan for the future—financially and otherwise—you'll have less anxiety and stress.

- Pursue goals. According to the *Age Erasers* books, "Goals prevent boredom, and that's important because boredom can put you at higher risk for disease, says Howard Friedman, Ph.D., professor of psychology and community medicine at the University of California, Riverside."

- Make your own decisions, "even if you need to rely on others' expertise or physical assistance to carry them out," advises *Live Longer, Live Better*. Few things are more likely to create a feeling of control than making your own decisions about your life.

Two of the most important aspects of control deserve their own headings: controlling your financial status and raising your understanding of the world around you. And so:

INCOME

Does wealth bring longevity? The signals are mixed—but, generally speaking, the answer is yes.

"While money may not buy happiness, higher income and higher social/economic status are unmistakably associated with a longer life span," Moore says. Some proof:

- Chopra examined a 1970 study of men and women in their late 60s. He reported, "Seventy percent of the long-lived men said that their income was the same as or better than when they were 55; 60 percent of the short-lived said they were worse off. . . . Many more of the long-lived women were financially better off than they were at age 55; many more of the short-lived had grown poorer."

- Moore says that in one U.S. government study, "Death rates in the poorest families (those earning $8,000 a year or less) were 250 percent [greater] than [in] families prosperous enough to earn $65,000, or about twice the typical American family's income. Such differences in death rates for social class or income category have been observed in the United States and Europe for 150 years."

- Bellamy mentions studies from the 1920s and 1940s, covering people in Paris, London, and the United States, in which "death rate[s] from all causes [were] definitely proportional to the economic state of the [people studied]."

- And Moore notes, "All the ten richest nations of the world have achieved life expectancies of over 75 years. And none of the ten poorest rises above 50 years."

HOW IT HAPPENS

"Many people suppose that better medical care explains the longer life spans among the better educated and more prosperous," Moore says. "The available evidence, however, suggests this is probably not the case. Those with lower social and economic status consistently consume more medical care than the more prosperous—primarily because their health status is generally worse."

In what way is it worse?

- In *Biological Anthropology,* Stanley Garn, Ph.D., of the University of Michigan's Center for Human Growth & Development writes, "In the United States . . . affluent better-educated women are leaner than their less educated and less affluent peers," and a lean body is likely to be a long-lived one. "There are also SES [socio-economic status]-related differences in fatness . . . in men as well," Garn adds.

Moreover, writes Case Western Reserve University anthropologist

Cynthia Beall, "[the] use of alcohol and major tranquilizers . . . are all associated with . . . lower socioeconomic factors."

Finally, Moore says, "Those who achieve more successful biological and social adaptation"—that is, the people who can prosper— "are experiencing lower long-term levels of stress."

But like all rules, the principle of "money equals longevity" has an exception or two.

HOLES IN THE THEORY

Moore points out, "Hong Kong, Spain, and Greece . . . have achieved a better life expectancy with only one-third the per-capita income of the United States. The economies of the former Communist countries of Hungary and Czechoslovakia out-performed the democracies of Spain and Greece, but their life expectancy trailed far behind."

Hayflick adds, "Ninety percent of American centenarians have an annual income of less than five thousand dollars, not counting food stamps, federal payments to nursing homes, or in-kind support from family and friends."

A CONCLUSION

Income may not be a central make-or-break factor in determining how long people live, but there is at least as much evidence in favor of a prosperous life as there is for a cash-poor one.

And most people would rather be rich than poor.

LEARNING

As the first part of this book noted, the profile of the long-lived person includes intelligence and education.

Like a good income, a well-trained mind can help to keep you relaxed and confident. The more that you know about anything that you need to know—from medical knowledge to how to fix plumbing—the more secure and confident you'll feel.

Staying Young, the *Age Erasers* books, *Live Longer, Live Better*, and Bortz's *Dare to Be 100* list various ways to build up your intelligence and education. Among the most common:

- Take up new challenges. They'll stimulate your mind.

- Listen to different viewpoints and sources of information.

- Exercise. Working out increases alertness, memory, and other tools that build an educated mind.

- Stay sociable; spend plenty of time with people. You'll inevitably learn things that you couldn't find out by being alone.

- When you're learning something new, don't rush it. Take your time. Rushing can build anxiety, which can block learning.

- Follow your heart and do activities that you enjoy. If you like doing something, you'll probably be eager to find out how to do it better.

- Develop new skills. (Many experts recommend learning to speak a foreign language.) If you master something that you've never tried before, you'll feel confident about handling other challenges.

Building the brain isn't necessarily easy, but it can unquestionably pay off. Ronald Klatz, M.D. (president of the American Longevity Research Institute), and Robert Goldman, M.D. (cofounder of the American Academy of Anti-Aging Medicine), put it clearly in their book *Stopping the Clock: Why Many of Us Will Live Past 100—And Enjoy Every Minute*: "The most powerful anti-aging weapon that you have is your mind."

WORKERS LIVE LONGER. A UNIVERSITY OF GEORGIA STUDY OF centenarians reported that they recommended work above all other secrets to long life. Productive activity is typical of people who age in a healthy way.

- Citing a survey of Soviet gerontological research conducted by Soviet longevity authority Dimitri Chebotarev, Georgakas says, "The longevous tend to work continually throughout their lives."

- Chopra notes that in the Caucasus, where there are more centenarians per thousand people than in most other places in the world, people typically work even into their 80s for several hours a day.

- "Women with demanding jobs have a lower risk of heart attack than women who don't work. The reason may be that they have more of a sense of control over their lives, a feeling linked to a lower illness rate," says *Live Longer, Live Better.*

- "In a study of 1,200 centenarians, Osborn Segerberg, Jr. reported that 'hard work' was the most frequent reason given for living so long. A whopping 89 percent said they'd worked hard all their lives," reports journalist Sue Browder in *Woman's Day* magazine.

CHALLENGING OR CONGENIAL?

A happy worker may be a long-lived worker.

- Browder notes that in Segerberg's study of centenarians, "Successful agers work hard, and *enjoy* it. . . . Studies consistently show that people who work hard *and hate it* are more likely to get certain types of cancer."

- Georgakas refers to a survey of more than 400 Americans over age 95, saying, "these nonagenarians . . . worked at jobs they liked."

- *Live Longer, Live Better,* noting that orchestra conductors tend to live long lives, observes, "Researchers link the maestros' longevity to their sense of being in control of their lives and the enjoyment of their work."

Enjoyable work isn't necessarily easy work. "The work of the longevous is physically demanding," Georgakas reports, based on Chebotarev's findings. The long-living people of the Caucasus, Georgakas adds, "enjoyed physical labor so much that they would have been as angry at being denied the right to work as they had [been] when landlords forced them to work."

So if you genuinely enjoy digging ditches or toting bales, go to it.

OCCUPATIONS

There is not much consensus as to the jobs that are likeliest to lead to long life. But there are some general trends.

The benefits of success

Winners may live long. As George Washington University's Moore writes in *Life Span*, "Longevity advantages flow to individuals capable of prospering within the confining but substantial demands of modern technical society."

For instance:

- *Biological Anthropology* notes that educated white-collar workers are less likely to develop osteoarthritis than others. "In both the United States and Europe, white-collar professionals have longer average life spans than those with lower-skilled jobs," says Moore.

- Leaders tend to outlive followers. Moore notes that among discharged veterans of the armed services, officers have had lower death rates than noncommissioned officers, who have had lower death rates than privates. He also cites a survey of white ministers that revealed that their chances of dying prematurely were about half that of other white men. In *How and Why We Age*, Hayflick notes that popes outlive the general population, cites a 19-year survey in which "the rate of death in the entire group of [orchestra] conductors was [found to be] 38 percent below that of the general population," and adds that in a Metropolitan Life Insurance study, "Top executives outlived others at all lower levels of accomplishment in business."

But before you go for a management training course, consider the following:

Jobs don't cause longevity; long-living people get good jobs

Hayflick points out that the people in supposedly life-lengthening jobs were set up to live long even before they got the jobs. "Do popes live longer than the general population? Yes, but only because the data is biased. The group that popes were chosen from represents the most vigorous survivors of a younger and larger qualified group."

Moore adds that their jobs may not be giving popes, generals, and company presidents long lives. Instead, the traits that enable people to get such jobs—rather than the jobs themselves—may encourage longevity. He says, "It is . . . possible those with more education and ability are taking conscious steps to prolong their lives, taking actions seen less frequently among those with less education, lower intelligence, or less-skilled jobs. Increased rates of smoking, alcohol abuse, drug abuse, and obesity have all been observed among those with low social/economic status."

The good news for people who aren't in white-collar jobs or leadership positions is that their jobs don't necessarily force them into short lives. Since anyone can "take conscious steps to prolong their lives"—exercising, eating healthy, reducing stress—anyone, regardless of his or her job, can live as long as an orchestra conductor or pope.

Workplaces

One place where jobs do affect longevity is in factories.

"Irrefutable research has established the link between cancers and working with substances like vinyl chloride, asbestos, industrial dyes, chromates, nickel, uranium, and glass fibers," says Georgakas. He adds, "The linkage of black lung with coal mining and brown lung with textile weaving is . . . beyond scientific dispute."

In any workplace, blue-collar or otherwise, another potential source of incapacity and death is falling. The Occupational Safety and Health Administration (OSHA) notes that stairs, ladders, girders, stages and other places with more than one level are prime spots for accidents.

To prevent falls, the *Age Erasers* books advise wearing safety gear where the job requires it and checking workplaces for anything on which you can trip, slip, or fall. Finally, "[find the person] whose job it is to make detailed reports of accidents to insurance companies, safety committees, and workers compensation . . . then ask where and when every injury took place during the past twelve months. Then make sure you don't fall into the same traps."

If that doesn't work, look for a new job. Georgakas sums it up: "Where such clear and present dangers exist in the workplace, pro-longevous persons have no option but to switch to other industries."

RETIREMENT

Most experts believe that traditional retirement is not helpful for longevity.

"For centuries in Abkhazia [a region of the Caucasus with a high longevity rate], sedentary retirement was unknown except in cases of disability," Chopra says. He also cites a 1973 study in New York of 79 healthy people 87 years of age and older that found "the majority did not retire early."

"The longevous are atypical humans in their adamant refusal to retire from work, even when they are financially able," says Georgakas. "Longevous persons never truly retire. Either they have chosen jobs that do not require it, or they shift to new activities that are just as physically and intellectually demanding as their former work had been."

Why? How does lifelong work build a long life?

The dangers of retirement

Retirement can kill. "There is a high death rate in the years immediately following retirement," says Georgakas.

Chopra explains, "In the first few years after retirement, heart attack and cancer rates soar, and early death overtakes men who were otherwise healthy before they retired. Early retirement death, as the syndrome is called, depends on the perception that one's useful days are over; this is only a perception, but for someone who holds it firmly, it is enough to cause disease and death."

Live Longer, Live Better lists retirement itself as a strong source of stress, almost equal to that of being fired from work.

Changing retirement into a life extender

If the active life is a long one, the passive life is a killer. "One way people age themselves," the *Chicago Tribune*'s Gorner and Kotulak write in *Aging On Hold*, "is to view retirement as a time for reduced activity. That can lead to weakness and debilitation."

To avoid that trap, plan ahead. As Stanford's Walter Bortz writes in *Dare to Be 100*, "Without planning and anticipation, there is often an overwhelming and acute depression, coupled with inaction."

Among the areas for planning:

- Health care. With retirement comes time for exercise and other ways to improve health. "Health is your own job, and retirement often gives you the chance to take even better care of yourself," says Bortz.

- Money. Make sure that you have enough for a long active life. Says Bortz, "Lack of financial resources is debilitating to morale—it leads to major health problems."

- Living arrangements. Many people change homes when they retire. That's not necessarily a bad thing. As Bortz says, "Several research studies show a strong correlation between longevity and satisfaction with living arrangements."

But he dislikes the idea of moving to a new community upon retirement. "The loss of continuity with home, family, and community is dangerous."

If you do choose to replant yourself, *Staying Young* suggests, "Visit in the off-season. . . . Ask local residents what they think are the most problematic challenges of the area. . . . Make a recreational checklist and see if the area meets your needs. . . . Look for like-minded people . . . [and] survey medical-care facilities."

- Work. Retirement needn't mean idleness. Bortz says, "Retirement provides the opportunity to rethink work." You can "retire" by shifting from full-time work to something that leaves time for other activities. Bortz mentions such options as "job sharing, flexible scheduling, seasonal employment, and other creative opportunities."

  There's precedent for this setup among the long-lived hard-working people of the Caucasus. "Older workers shortened their hours in the fields as they approached 80 and 90; instead of laboring for 10 to 15 hours, they might quit after three to five hours," says Chopra.

  Whatever you decide, Stanford University's James Fries writes in *Living Well*, "You should seriously reevaluate [your choice] at least every five years." In *Reversing Human Aging*, Michigan State's Michael Fossel suggests, "You might alternate working and 'retiring,' coming back to a job, or beginning a new one, every few decades."

Too many options? *Live Longer, Live Better* advises, "If you're not sure of your retirement goals, you may want to try a retirement rehearsal by taking a leave of absence from your job. Another option might be to settle into retirement in stages by going from full-time to part-time work."

SLEEP HAS FIGURED IN LONGEVITY FOR MILLENNIA. HAYFLICK SAYS, "A Babylonian epic, carved into twelve clay tablets around 650 B.C., describes Gilgamesh's obsession with immortality. Gilgamesh, a ruler in southern Mesopotamia who lived around the year 3000 B.C., consults with a sage who tells him that to be victorious over death, he must first conquer sleep by staying awake for seven days and nights. Gilgamesh tries and fails."

Search for Immortality adds, "In ancient Greek myth, the shepherd boy Epimenides fell asleep for fifty-seven years while looking for a lost sheep; in the Norse sagas, the Valkyrie Brunhild slumbered inside a circle of fire until she was awakened by Siegfried, the only man brave enough to pierce the flames. The princess Sleeping Beauty, heroine of the seventeenth-century French fairy tale, dozed for 100 years before a prince revived her with a kiss. Nineteenth-century American author Washington Irving brought the theme to modern times with the tale of Rip Van Winkle, a New York villager of the 1770s who cavorted one night with a ghostly crew of mountain spirits, fell into a deep slumber, and awakened some twenty years later."

Sleeping for decades is unlikely. Hayflick says, "The idea of increasing longevity by extending sleep has been limited to the imagination of fiction writers."

Nevertheless, sleep can aid the body in reaching for a long life. "Invariably, longevous people report lifelong patterns of regular and satisfying sleep," Georgakas says.

Besides, if you lack regular and satisfying sleep, you die. *Dr. Bob Arnot's Guide to Turning Back the Clock* observes, "Chronic lack of sleep reduces your life expectancy."

HOW DOES SLEEP WORK?

THE BENEFITS OF SLEEP

While you're out cold, your body works. "During sleep, your body . . . can devote itself to healing," *Staying Young* explains. The *Age Erasers* books say, "The body releases its greatest concentration of growth hormone—the substance that helps our bodies repair damaged tissue—during sleep."

THE EFFECTS OF SLEEPLESSNESS

The major ones are:

- Lack of immunity. "Without enough rest, your immune system will suffer," say the *Age Erasers* books. In *18 Natural Ways to Look and Feel Half Your Age,* Norman Ford explains, "The natural killer cells of the immune system fail to adequately defend the body against cancer and infectious disease."

- Accidents. Arnot says, "Lack of sleep is one of the leading causes of loss of life from industrial and automobile accidents." Ford agrees: "One survey showed that young adults who were sleep-deficient had as many traffic accidents as drunk drivers."

- Stress. Without sufficient sleep, Ford notes, "Both men and women lose energy and vigor and become morose, irritable, forgetful, confused, listless, hostile and impatient."

HOW MUCH SLEEP DO YOU NEED?

The consensus of the authorities ranges from six to ten hours per night, with the plurality recommending seven to eight hours.

- In a UCLA study of more than 6,000 people, the long-lived among them had a habit of sleeping seven or eight hours per night.

- "Men who report fewer than four hours of sleep per night have about three times higher the likelihood of dying within six years, compared with those who sleep seven to eight hours per night," reports *The American Geriatrics Society's Complete Guide to Aging & Health.*

- Joyce Walsleben, Ph.D., of New York University's Sleep Disorder Center says, "People who sleep less than six hours or more than ten hours have a higher mortality rate."

EXCEPTIONS

Many people, of course, can make do with less sleep than others. Georgakas adds, "There is such a wide variation in sleeping needs that it is best to ask not how long one has slept but how well." Waking up in the middle of the night, sleep apnea (disturbances in breathing), and other problems diminish the quality of sleep. If you suffer from sleep disturbances, see a doctor.

Quantity does matter over the long term. Bortz notes, "It is true that many of us can go months and even years on four to five hours a night, but the deficit is cumulative." In other words, going without sleep will catch up with you.

But sleeping a little less may not hurt much. As Hayflick points out, "When you are asleep . . . you are not living life in any way comparable to the way you live it when you are awake. . . . [Therefore,] extending longevity becomes a question of increasing one's waking hours. . . . If, for example, you set your alarm clock for 30 minutes less sleep each night from age 25 to age 60, you would gain about 266 days in additional waking hours, or 'life.'"

Hayflick stops short of recommending less sleep per night. But if you are already sleeping eight hours per night and find that you can use an extra half hour of waking time, it probably won't hurt your overall longevity to get up 30 minutes early.

SLEEP IN THE LATER YEARS

Age may cause variations in the amount of sleep that people need. Or it may not. The longevity experts disagree.

"We need less sleep as we grow older," Fries says. "The eight hours a day that are appropriate for the young adult decrease to seven in our sixties and to six or less in our seventies and beyond."

In *Earl Mindell's Anti-Aging Bible*, Pacific Western University professor Mindell counters, "There are many myths about sleep, and one of the most prevalent is that the older you get, the less sleep you need. In reality, the experts say, if you needed eight hours of sleep at 20 years of age, you still require the same amount of sleep at 40 or even at 80."

And Bortz is in the middle. "Some older people seem to need more sleep, others less."

Sleep, like many other aspects of human life, varies from person to person. If you think that you're getting too much or too little sleep, check with your doctor.

THE SLEEPING ROOM

Arnot says, "Make your bedroom a vault"—protected from anything that can interfere with a good night's sleep.

Most experts recommend that the room be quiet, dark, and comfortable. But some authorities note, in Arnot's words, that "some [people] need a level of ambient background noise." These noises can include low levels of auto traffic, air conditioner hums, ocean roars, or soft music.

Other important factors for the bedroom:

- Temperature. While many experts recommend a slightly cool room, others allow temperatures up to 80 degrees. Perhaps the best way to reconcile the difference is to heed Arnot's advice: "You're the best measure of too hot, not the thermostat. If you feel too hot, it's too hot."

- The sacredness of the bedchamber. The American Geriatrics Society says, "Avoid using the bedroom for activities that are not conducive to sleep. This will serve to keep the bed as a powerful stimulus to sleep." As Michael Vitiello, Ph.D., of the University of Washington's Sleep and Aging Research Program says "If you introduce activities like paying bills, eating pizza, and watching television [into the bedroom], the body gets confused and may not want to sleep in bed."

A SCHEDULE FOR SLEEP

Sleep on schedule. If you don't, you could risk contracting life-shortening diseases. *Staying Young* says, "Eight out of ten people who switch back and forth between day and night shifts have sleep problems, reports the *New England Journal of Medicine*, and they have more heart disease and digestive disorders than people with normal sleep patterns."

To arrange for regular sleep patterns, keep other aspects of life on a regular schedule. Arnot quotes Walsleben as follows: "Meals at regular times and all activities, like exercising, at predictable times will strengthen the wake system to be awake when you want to be and help calm you down when it's time for the sleep system."

Other activities that affect sleep:

GETTING UP AT A REGULAR TIME

"Going to bed and waking up at the same time every day," the *Age Erasers* books advise, "will condition your internal clock so that you will fall asleep easier, sleep more soundly, and wake feeling refreshed."

Sleeping late on weekends, though tempting, isn't healthy. As *Staying Young* notes, "Sleeping late . . . throws off your biological clock." Arnot explains, "Every extra hour you sleep requires a full 24 hours to reset. If you get up at 7 A.M. weekdays and 10 A.M. Sunday, it'll be Wednesday before your body is back on track."

AWAKENING EARLY

Early rising may or may not aid sleep, but it does seem to be a part of longevity. G. M. Humphry, a turn-of-the-century doctor who examined hundreds of people age 90 and up found that the majority of his patients rose early. So did 79 people age 87 and above whom psychiatrist Stephen Jewett examined in 1973.

Early rising may not actually cause longevity, of course. Work is typically a part of long life, and people who work hard may rise early to get their work done. So early rising may be only incidental to living long—but the facts remain: many long-lived people have the habit of getting up early.

AFTERNOON NAPPING

"People's alertness and ability to perform tasks drop during the midafternoon," says *Live Longer, Live Better*. "The urge to sleep in the middle of the day appears to be natural."

Natural, yes; healthy, maybe not.

Afternoon naps can worsen nighttime sleep, according to several authorities. "Very often, some of the more severe symptoms [of sleep disorders], such as chronic insomnia, may be caused by . . . something as simple as too much daytime napping," Mindell says.

A minority disagrees. Timothy Monk, Ph.D., of the University of Pittsburgh School of Medicine says, "Many individuals who don't get all the sleep they need at night benefit from a short siesta in the afternoon."

How to choose between the anti-nap and pro-nap advocates? The *Age Erasers* books offer some sensible advice: "If napping makes you feel good the rest of the day, if it doesn't interfere with your evening sleep, and if your schedule permits, by all means take a siesta when you feel that afternoon slump."

That's a lot of ifs. Here's one more. If you do take a nap, advise several experts, keep it under an hour (some experts go as short as half an hour). As *Staying Young* explains, "Longer [naps] will keep you from feeling sleepy at bedtime"—and bedtime is exactly when you *should* feel sleepy.

EXERCISING

Workouts are good for sleep. "Daily exercise can leave you properly tuckered out at night," Mindell explains. Fries even calls exercise "the most important promoter of deep sleep."

Keep in mind, though, that workouts can make you energetic. As the *Age Erasers* books testify, "[they] keep you awake for quite a while." So, in the words of *Live Longer*, "Don't exercise vigorously just before bedtime."

Instead, say many experts, work out at least two hours before bedtime.

LATE DINING

Another thing to do at least two hours before bed: Stop eating. If you eat, "your rumbling stomach may keep you up for hours or may make your sleep less refreshing," the *Age Erasers* books explain.

Some foods are more troublesome than others. The *Age Erasers* books note, "Don't eat a full meal, spicy foods, or a Dagwood sandwich less than three hours before bedtime." And Arnot says, "Too much roughage can also cause a poor night's sleep by keeping your intestines at work, so avoid too much steak, bran, and raw vegetables at dinnertime."

However, the *Age Erasers* books allow, "A small snack before bed is okay."

FRETTING

For proper sleep, Michael Vitiello advises, "Get your troubles out of your system. Don't use the bed as a setting for anxiety." To avoid this problem, get your bill paying, planning for tomorrow, and worrying done at least two hours before bed.

DRINKING

Since frequent trips to the bathroom can keep you up all night, it's a good idea to stop drinking anything at least two hours before bed.

But some beverages are good for sleep, and some are bad. For example:

- If you consume coffee—and, for that matter, chocolate, soft drinks, or other caffeinated foods—stop early. Although Ryback permits stopping as late as 4 P.M., several other experts believe that noon is a better safer time to quit.

  Why so soon? Caffeine can stay in the bloodstream for six hours or more.

  Arnot admits, though, "This response is quite individual. Some men can drink a cup right before they go to bed and sleep just fine." And Fries concedes that the duration of caffeine's power can shift: "As you grow older, all drugs last longer in your body."

- Alcohol may put you to sleep but not leave you there. Citing the work of Quentin Regestein, M.D., of the Brigham and Women's Hospital Sleep Clinic, Arnot says that alcohol "disturbs sleep by stimulating production of adrenaline-like neurotransmitters [brain chemicals], interfering with breathing and increasing the need to urinate."

  "It also makes you more prone to nighttime awakenings," Mindell says. Once awake, says Ryback, you may not be able to get back to sleep. What's worse, "even if you spend many hours asleep, they probably won't be good hours, and you'll feel rotten in the morning," say the *Age Erasers* books.

  So avoid alcohol before bed.

- Better for sleep than coffee or alcohol is tea.

  Mindell says, "Chamomile tea has a relaxing effect on the body and is an old-time cure for insomnia." But, he cautions, "Chamomile is a member of the daisy family, which also includes ragweed. If you are allergic to any members of the daisy family, avoid this herb."

  Other sleep-inducing teas include Siberian ginseng, skullcap, valerian, lemon balm, and peppermint, says Mindell.

  Since caffeine can interfere with sleep, it's a good idea to avoid it in tea.

- It's an old prescription, and it works: Warm milk can help you sleep. Milk, Ryback notes, "contains the relaxing amino acid tryptophan," which can aid sleep.

RELAXING

If you shouldn't eat, drink, exercise, or worry before bed, what should you do?

Unwind. Take a bath, listen to music, read a magazine, walk the dog, or do anything else that you find restful.

It's a good idea to do your presleep activities as regularly as any others. Following the same pattern night after night can be soothing and can ease you into slumber.

TRANQUILIZERS

Unless your doctor prescribes them, don't use them.

"Sleeping pills will work at first, but then you adapt to them and you're worse off than before," says Ryback. "You become dependent on the pills even though they start losing their effectiveness."

Even when they work, tranquilizers may cause trouble. "Although they can help put you to sleep, they can also interfere with your natural sleeping patterns and actually cause you to have a less restful night," report the *Age Erasers* books. As *Staying Young* explains, "These drugs decrease the amount of deep quality sleep. So while you may get to sleep sooner, your sleep is poorer."

Finally, Mindell warns, "Barbiturates can be habit forming and can cause dangerous interactions with other medications."

WHEN TO GO TO SLEEP?

"Go to bed sufficiently early so that you wake up naturally each morning without an alarm," Ford advises.

It's best if, at a "sufficiently early" hour, you're actually tired enough to sleep. Slipping into bed when you're not tired will simply lead to lying there wide awake.

"Don't lie awake in bed for more than 20 minutes," says *Live Longer*. If you do, the *Age Erasers* books say, "you'll only condition yourself not to fall asleep while you're there."

Finally—and to no surprise— "keep a regular time for going to bed," Ryback advises. "When you do go to sleep at a regular time, not only will you fall asleep more readily, but the sleep you get will be more restful."

GETTING TO SLEEP

Does falling asleep, something that you do at least once a day, actually require a technique?

It can, if you have a hard time getting to sleep. If you do . . .

"When you get into bed, don't even think about sleeping," advises *Staying Young*. "Instead, relax for 15 to 20 minutes by reading or listening to music or using relaxation techniques, meditation, or prayer."

Fries offers advice that is more general but perhaps more useful: "Develop for yourself the routines that work best."

Perhaps the most popular presleep activity is sex.

"Sex is a natural relaxant that helps soothe the body and promote a good night's sleep," Mindell says. "Dr. Regestein [of the Brigham and Women's Hospital Sleep Clinic] believes that, like a hot bath or anything else that reduces tension, [sex] will help."

For more about sex, see the next section of this book.

OVER MANY CENTURIES, *SEARCH FOR IMMORTALITY* REPORTS, "HUMAN sexual energy was understandably viewed as a potent force for rejuvenation."

Take Taoism. "Taoism extolled ritualized sexual practices as a key to long life," explains *Search for Immortality*. "A male Taoist adept was enjoined to practice coitus reservatus, always stopping short of his own orgasm while bringing his partner to a climax. The semen thus held in check was thought to invigorate and rejuvenate the man's entire system."

"The great Dutch physician Boerhaave (1668–1738)," says Hayflick, "recommended an old burgomaster of Amsterdam to lie between two young girls, assuring him that he would recover strength and spirits."

Does sex really extend life?

THE STATISTICS

Yes, sex really does extend life.

- Researcher Maurice Ernest, working in the 1930s, surveyed historical records from Roman times onward. Among Ernest's conclusions for longevity: "Enjoy a reasonable sex life."

- People who reach old age often have healthy sex drives. Georgakas reports: "One study, conducted by Duke University, which covered over 200 men and women between the ages of 60 and 94 disclosed that 50 percent of them were enjoying sexual relations. Among octogenarians, the rate was between 10 and 20 percent, with many [others] stating that it was the lack of suitable partners rather than the lack of desire which prevented them from being sexually active."

- Sexual activity releases endorphins (brain chemicals that reduce stress). Ford adds, "The strong social bonding and human contact of lovemaking—with its loving, touching, hugging, and warmth—

boosts the health of every cell and organ in the body. A climax is a splendid muscle relaxant and stress reliever, and it strengthens the competence of the immune system."

THE CELIBACY CONUNDRUM

As noted earlier, popes—who are, by reputation at least, celibate—tend to outlive the general population. So did the members of the 19th-century religious sect the Shakers, who practiced celibacy and averaged a life expectancy of 67 years, "while that of the rest of the population was merely 47," according to *Search for Immortality*.

But everyone who has ever become a Shaker or a pope has done so as an adult. "The Shakers," says *Search for Immortality*, "had therefore already survived childhood, whereas a high infant mortality rate necessarily lowered the average life expectancy in the general population." The same is true for popes, but more so, since most popes attain that high office at an age when many other people are already dead.

So you don't have to avoid sex to live as long as a pope or a Shaker. That these long-lived people are celibate seems to be a coincidence.

LEGENDS OF SEX

Is there any aspect of human life that has generated more misinformation than sex?

Two myths involving longevity and sex are:

SEX KILLS

The jokes about men dying because sex was too hard for their heart are merely legends. According to *Live Longer, Live Better*, "The likelihood that sexual intercourse will cause [a heart] attack is extremely slight. In fact, research shows that sexually active heart attack patients enjoy a reduced risk of future heart attacks."

In other words, sex has few physical risks, and just about any adult can enjoy it and get longevity benefits from it. Hayflick advises, "Remember the three stages of sexual activity: triweekly, try weekly, and try weakly—but do try."

OLD PEOPLE DON'T HAVE SEX

Oh, yes, they do. A 1995 survey conducted for *Parade* magazine revealed that among people age 65 and older, 40 percent have sex more than twice a month (on average).

"Physical changes do occur as you age," *Staying Young* explains, "but none of them need undermine the pleasures of a couple's sex life. In fact, many older people maintain that sex is *better* in later years because there are no worries about pregnancy, no children nearby, and no pressures of work."

CONTACT WITH OTHERS

HAVING CLOSE FRIENDSHIPS, A FAMILY, A MARRIAGE, AND OTHER relationships can help you live longer.

- "In a study of 2,754 people in Tecumseh, Michigan, men who donated their time to community organizations were two and a half times less likely to die from all types of disease than their non-involved peers," writes health journalist Sue Browder.

- "Studies have shown that connected people have less than half the mortality rates as lonely people, and the closer the relationship, the more powerful the survival effect," Bortz says.

- Georgakas reports research showing that nuns, who live in communal settings, have had better-than-average life spans.

- The *Age Erasers* books report: "One of the first studies linking relationships and longevity took place in Alameda County, California. Researchers there found that over a nine-year period, the people with the strongest social and community ties were the least likely to die. Not surprisingly, the most isolated people had the highest death rate. Three more studies have duplicated these findings: in each study, people who were isolated were three to five times more likely to die than people who had intimate relationships."

- The *Age Erasers* books refer to Redford Williams, M.D., of Duke University Medical Center: "His team followed 1,368 heart disease patients for nine years. . . . Dr. Williams says, 'Patients with neither a spouse nor a friend were three times more likely to die than those involved in a caring relationship.'"

The next sections cover the major types of close relationships and their effect on longevity.

LIVING WITH LOVED ONES

Don't live alone. Chopra notes the research of Harvard psychologist George Vaillant: "The longest-lived individuals, he believed, are . . . rarely living alone."

"By far the most prolongevous living arrangement," says Georgakas, "is a multigenerational household or community." He adds, "The companionship aspect of living arrangements is underscored by findings that feelings of loneliness often precede death."

The best companions for long life are spouses, relatives, and pets.

MARRIAGE

A happy marriage extends life. The proof stretches over the centuries.

- "Excess mortality has . . . been observed among the unmarried, widowed, divorced, and separated. It was identified among members of the European nobility in the fifteenth century and confirmed in an 1848 study of French society," writes Moore.

- Georgakas reports one of the findings of G. M. Humphry's turn-of-the-century study of 900 nonagenarians: "Over two-thirds of the women had been married."

- The University of Wales's Bellamy, in *Ageing: A Biomedical Perspective,* mentions a study of Americans in the 1940s: "The mortality of single persons, and especially of the divorced and widowed, was definitely higher than [that] of married couples." Tuberculosis, for example, killed divorced men at a rate more than three times, and widowed men at more than four times, that of married men. Divorced white men had the highest death rate, with twice the chance of dying than any married persons.

- In the 1960s, the Soviet Union's Gerontological Institute of Kiev interviewed 40,000 people over age 80. The survey found that 99 percent of the men questioned had been married; so had 97 percent of the women.

- A 1970s study of 294 centenarians in the Caucasus revealed that almost all had been married for most if not all of their adult lives.

- Today, says Georgakas, "in the United States, at every age past 20, death rates are lower for those who are married than those who are single, widowed, or divorced, the mortality for unmarried men living alone being the highest." Specifically, single men live, on average, about a decade less than married men, according to the National Center for Health Statistics.

How marriage lengthens life
Married people, according to the *Age Erasers* books, drink less alcohol, eat less junk food, and exercise more regularly than single people. They're more relaxed and fall ill less often.

The *Age Erasers* books, citing the views of psychologist Vicki Helgeson of Carnegie Mellon University, report that heart-attack victims who can talk honestly with their spouses about the attack are less likely to have chest pains or be readmitted to the hospital within a year than are victims without a spouse.

Even a bad marriage can be good—among men, at least. "For men, the quality of married life doesn't seem to matter," says *Age Erasers for Women*. "Their health seems to improve even if they're in a wretched marriage."

Happy marriage

For both men and women, a good marriage seems more life-prolonging than a bad one. "The longevity factor . . . does not appear to be marriage itself so much as living in a situation that provides companionship and feelings of self-esteem," Georgakas says. "Longevous individuals frequently say that successful marriages are the secret of their long lives."

The *Age Erasers* books, again referring to the work of Carnegie Mellon University's Helgeson, report that for men or women, conflict and hostility within a marriage can raise blood pressure and debilitate the immune system.

A happy marriage is especially important for women. Psychologist Robert Levenson of the University of California at Berkeley says, "A woman's health seems to follow the health of the relationship. . . . If the marriage is satisfying, then [her] health seems to be good. If [she's] in an unsatisfying marriage, [her] health suffers."

Exactly how a happy marriage extends life is not clear, but Moore offers a clue: "While marriage apparently does have inherent value to health, it is also an important marker for successful biological and social adjustment. And those who make the most successful adjustments to the pressures and demands of life will live the longest."

Chopra notes that Harvard psychologist George Vaillant, who tracked American men from the 1940s through the 1980s, came to a similar conclusion. "The longest-lived individuals, he believed, are also the best adapted in their psychological life, a state characterized by . . . regarding their marriages as satisfying."

It may sound too good to be true—a well-adjusted person will have both a happy marriage and a long life—but true it appears to be. The sections of this book on training the mind may help put you on the road to a well-adjusted way of living.

FAMILY LIFE

Families can drive you mad, but they can also nurture longevity. Among long-lived people, Georgakas says, "The overwhelming majority have lived the greater part of their lives in a family unit."

He notes, for instance, that among the long-lived people of the Caucasus, "all lived with their families." And he mentions a Soviet study by Russian longevity expert Dimitri Chebotarev that revealed that "the longest living often remain in the same village or region as their parents and relatives."

Family seems especially important in helping overcome problems of the mind, emotion, and psyche. Ryback mentions "family closeness" as a means of reducing stress. And Chopra notes that laid-off Michigan auto workers, who have sustained their health due to the closeness of friends, also received strong health-nurturing support from their families.

The exception

Despite the advantages of family, not all families are conducive to long life. "Weight problems are especially common among people who grew up in households that were somewhat dysfunctional," Cornell University's Aronne writes in *Weigh Less, Live Longer*. "Even in happy homes, attitudes about food can create weight problems. For example, if food was a sign of togetherness, eating may be the way that you comfort yourself with memories of your youth."

But for the most part, a family that is close both emotionally and physically is good for long life.

PETS

The presence of an animal can extend life.

- "Taking care of a pet has been shown to help reduce blood pressure, heart rate, and stress levels," notes *Live Longer, Live Better.*

- "One study of 5,741 people in Melbourne, Australia, showed that pet owners had lower levels of blood pressure and cholesterol than nonowners," report the *Age Erasers* books.

- "According to one study, heart patients who owned pets had a higher survival rate one year after their hospitalization than those who didn't," says *Live Longer, Live Better.*

- "Research has demonstrated that a pet dog can be an even better stress buster than a human friend in certain situations," reports *Staying Young.*

"Although all sorts of companion animals have been shown to have therapeutic effects, dogs do seem to have an edge," say the *Age Erasers* books.

In a UCLA study of elderly people mourning the death of a loved one, the people who owned pets apparently felt healthier than the ones without pets; the people who had no pets saw their doctors 16 percent more often than pet owners did and 20 percent more than dog owners in particular. The relationship with a pet may have provided a sense of companionship and even nurturing—and walking the dogs provided exercise.

As Bortz puts it, "The intimacy of a soft head, a warm tongue, and a wagging tail is strong medicine indeed. In the final analysis, a pet is a fine doctor and a dear friend."

COMMUNITIES

Where people respect the aged, the aged live longer.

- "Exceptionally long-lived survivors invariably occur in small isolated communities where life-style and the social role of the elderly favor long life," says Bellamy. "Often, the aged in these communities have a high social status."

- Georgakas paraphrases Russian longevity expert Dimitri Chebotarev: "The longevous are most highly concentrated where local tradition demands respect for elders."

- "In societies where old age is accepted as part of the social fabric, elders remain extremely vigorous—lifting, climbing, and bending in ways that we do not accept as normal in our elderly," Chopra says.

But not all places for the elderly are good for the elderly.

OLD FOLKS' HOMES

Institutions, retirement communities, nursing homes—many people live there, but such places don't usually extend life.

"The least desirable of last homes is an institution where 5 percent or more of inhabitants are 65," says Bortz. "Institutionalization increases mortality two and one-half fold."

Two of the most common types of such living arrangements are retirement communities and nursing homes.

Retirement communities

In general, longevity experts don't recommend retirement communities. "Many popular retirement communities are overbuilt, congested, and expensive," says *Live Longer, Live Better*.

What's more, retirement communities—like other places where most of the people are aged—have a special disadvantage. "The loss of [a close] friend often leads to the early death of the survivor," Georgakas says.

"Retirement communities suffer from this phenomenon, as they are constantly recording deaths without having the full range of generations, which would include births, to redress the emotional balance."

Although living in a retirement community is probably less life-extending than living among family and friends of all ages, it's still better than living alone, especially if the community is well run. "Such communities have the advantage of keeping their inhabitants in touch with a wide social circle with many regularized community activities," Georgakas says. The American Geriatrics Society agrees: "Some individuals feel a sense of added security and peace of mind [in retirement communities]."

If you're not among those individuals, think hard before joining a retirement community.

Nursing homes

"[In] the usual nursing-home situation," Georgakas says, "dependency and abandonment are the rule." Dependency and abandonment are obviously the opposite of the close social contact and sense of control that can extend life.

Nursing homes may have medical problems, too. The American Geriatrics Society's guide warns that nursing homes may have "a lack of adequately trained staff, an inability of the nursing staff to administer intravenous therapy, [and] a lack of diagnostic services such as X rays."

Nursing homes may even help illnesses to spread. The American Geriatrics Society's guide notes, "In the nursing home, infection is the most common sudden medical problem leading to hospitalization." The problem with infections is simple and chilling, according to Peter Mayer of the State University of New York Health Science Center of Brooklyn. "Infectious diseases represent the second most frequent cause of death in the elderly of developed countries."

If a nursing home is necessary, *Live Longer*, Fries, and the American Geriatrics Society offer guidelines for choosing one:

- Visit the home often and at different times of day. Make sure that it's clean. See if the residents seem well cared for. Check for safety precautions, such as railings and grab bars. Find out what the food is like. Look for recreational space and planned activities and excursions.

- Ask if the staff has special training in long-term care and geriatrics. Look for a high ratio of nurses to residents. Make sure that a physician is on staff or at least on call.

- Ask for the home's Medicare and Medicaid certifications and/or state license. Read the latest annual state report on the home. Get referrals and recommendations from friends, relatives, doctors, and others who know the home.

- Make sure that the home is affordable. Find out how much of the cost is covered by insurance—and what will happen to a resident if the insurance money runs out.

- Make sure that the home's location and visiting hours are convenient for friends and relatives. Find out if it's close to a hospital.

Finally, people who live in nursing homes should have something to do and care about. As Chopra says, "Harvard psychologist Ellen Langer has demonstrated that people in nursing homes improve remarkably after altering their lives in the simplest ways—giving them a potted plant to tend, allowing them to make up their own menus, and taking charge of tidying their own rooms."

LEGENDS OF PLACES WITH MYSTICAL POWERS OF LONGEVITY ARE practically as old as the idea of longevity itself. The Garden of Eden is the most famous, but there are many others.

"Indian myths spoke of the far-off land of Utturakuru, where the magic tree of life grew," says Georgakas. He adds that islands of long life "figured in the mythology of Japan, Iran, and the Teutonic tribes."

The Greeks had many legends about places that bred long life. There was the mythical land of the Hyperboreans ("which literally means 'beyond the north wind,'" says Hayflick). Georgakas says the Greeks believed that longevity existed in the interior of Ethiopia and on an island or continent beyond the Strait of Gibraltar and in the mountains of Asia Minor.

The tradition continued to more recent times. "In 1498, Columbus claimed to have found the earthly paradise of immortality on the Venezuelan coast near the island of Trinidad," says Hayflick. And, of course, James Hilton's 1933 novel *Lost Horizon* described a land of long-lived people called Shangri-La.

FOUNTAINS OF YOUTH

Perhaps the most common legend of a place bestowing long life is that of a fountain of youth. "The fountain [of youth] theme is present in the histories of nearly every culture," says Fries.

"The earliest reference to rejuvenation by a fountain of youth can be found in Hindu writings dating from about 700 B.C.," Hayflick says. "References to rejuvenation by fountains also occur in the Old and New Testaments as well as in the Koran and Greek and Roman writings."

"The search for eternal youth is depicted in Roman mythology in the story of Jupiter transforming the nymph Juventas into a fountain of youth," reports *Live Longer, Live Better*. "Whoever bathed in her sweet-smelling waters became young and healthy."

Every schoolchild has learned of Juan Ponce de León's sixteenth-century search for a fountain of youth. "Ponce de León explored Bimini, Florida, and the Yucatán in his fruitless quest for immortality," says *Search for Immortality*. "He found death instead of youth, suffering a mortal wound in an Indian attack in 1521." He was about 61 years old.

THE REALITIES

"Maximum life span does vary geographically," says Bellamy. There are definite scientific clues as to the efficacy of some places as life lengtheners. But other claims are outright frauds.

JAPAN

To live a long time, live like the Japanese. "The Japanese," says Mindell, "have the longest life span of any nationality in the world." Depending on which source you consult, the average life span there is 79 or 80 years. Either number is higher than America's 76 years.

It's not a genetic advantage. "Japanese living in Japan have one set of cancers, but Japanese who have emigrated to the United States have another," says Georgakas. Moore reports on Japanese burial mounds, dating back more than 2,000 years, from which 236 skeletons were recovered. The bones revealed how long the people lived. "Life expectancy . . . was similar to that found in Cyprus or Morocco," says Moore. Since genes don't change much over the centuries, the Japanese of today still have the same genes that gave their ancestors lives no longer than those of the Cypriots or Moroccans.

If the advantage isn't genetic, what is it?

JAPANESE DIET

The experts credit food for at least part of Japanese longevity. Moore notes that the Japanese diet is low in calories: "Most [experts] think the

United States consumes too much at current levels of 3,600 calories a day. The long-lived Japanese consume 2,800 calories a day."

Moreover, Moore adds, "Japan has a diet very low in saturated fat and other animal products and low in fat of any kind."

Soybeans come in for the most praise. "The Japanese, who eat the most soybeans in the world—30 times more than Americans—live longer than anyone," says Carper in *Stop Aging Now!* Soybeans, she adds, fight cancer, keep arteries healthy, and strengthen bones.

Carper also praises the Japanese consumption of fish. "The Japanese," she says, "eat three times more fish than Americans." Fish is high in vitamins B_6, B_{12}, and D, as well as calcium and omega-3 fatty acids; it also lowers triglyceride levels.

"The traditional Japanese eat only small amounts of meat [and] poultry," says Arnot. He adds, "Fresh fruit is the dessert of choice." You don't have to be Japanese to know that cutting back on meat and eating fruit instead of sweets are a healthy way to go.

OTHER FACTORS

A minority view holds that culture is more important than diet. Moore observes that other long-lived peoples—the Swiss, for example, and the Greeks—include far more fat in their diets than the Japanese. "This suggests the longest life spans the world has ever known are compatible with [a variety of] dietary patterns, providing that nutrition is complete, abundant, and widely available."

Chopra adds that some Japanese immigrants to the United States "continued to have low rates of heart disease that did not correlate with diet." How did such people stay healthy? "[They] retained strong ties to Japanese culture despite their having moved to America," he says. "The various ways in which their awareness remained Japanese (by growing up in a Japanese neighborhood, attending school with other Japanese children, speaking their native language, and observing traditional customs and social ties) all contributed to producing healthy hearts."

DIET VERSUS CULTURE

Even if culture is more important than food, though, the traditional Japanese diet can help to extend life, and it can't hurt to try it. Besides, it's easier to adopt the Japanese diet than the entire Japanese culture.

But watch out; Japan is not perfect. The Japanese diet produces healthy hearts—but its "salty, smoked, and pickled foods combine to create Japan's two most serious health problems: stroke and stomach cancer," says Arnot.

Carper adds that for all of their health advantages, the Japanese tend to have high blood pressure. Arnot blames the high sodium in Japanese foods. He also condemns tempura ("which means batter-dipped and deep-fried"), egg dishes like *oyako-donburi,* and fried pork dishes like *tonkatsu.*

OKINAWA

If any place in the world encourages long life, it's this island. And the statistics prove it. The average life span for Okinawan women (who live a little longer than men) is the highest for anyone, male or female, in the world—more than 84 years, according an article by Deborah Franklin in *Health* magazine. "In Okinawa," Arnot adds, "more people live to age 100 than [in] any other place on Earth."

Including the rest of Japan. "Okinawa has two to forty times more centenarians than in any other part of Japan," says Bellamy. Carper says that Okinawans "have 30 to 40 percent less heart disease, stroke, cancer, diabetes, and age-related brain disease [than other Japanese]." "Many manage to postpone for decades, or avoid altogether, the . . . diseases that elsewhere tend to sap life before stealing it," notes the *Health* magazine article.

Most experts attribute these advantages to the food. Since the island has long been a crossroads "where traders from Asia and beyond couldn't help but swap recipes along with their luxury goods," says *Health,* the Okinawan diet has been more varied than that of the rest of Japan. The

Okinawans traditionally have eaten fruit, vegetables—especially soybeans—and seafood but have avoided salt and sugar, and Carper notes that they eat "17 to 40 percent fewer calories than other Japanese."

Although health journalist Carol Orlock admits, "the residents of Okinawa may be the beneficiaries of good genes—they may have inherited their longevity," the fact remains that the Okinawan diet is a healthy one that non-Okinawans can adopt. As *Health* states, "The island's life-enhancing [diet] should work just as well in Wichita or Warsaw."

THE CAUCASUS

The southern republics of the former Soviet Union—Georgia, Armenia, Abkhazia, Azerbaijan, Checheno-Ingush, and other areas in and near the Caucasus Mountains—are alleged to be home to some of the longest-lived people on Earth.

"According to American anthropologist Sula Benet, who spent several years studying the Caucasian people, they have been known for their longevity since ancient times," reports *Search for Immortality*. "Greek, Persian, and Arabian chronicles mention the long-lived peoples in the mountains between the Black and Caspian Seas."

In 1916, Georgakas reports, the Caucasian Essed Bey traveled the region and testified, "The Caucasian, on the average, will attain the age of 80 to 90 years. Centenarians and even older persons are by no means uncommon."

The reputation continues. Data from the census and other surveys put the number of centenarians at as much as 12 percent of the population. (In the United States, centenarians account for less than 1 percent of the population.)

Are the longevity claims true? Not all of them.

"Later investigations have failed to confirm [the] reputed longevities," says UCLA's Walford in *The Anti-Aging Plan*. And Hayflick says flatly, "Supercentenarian age claims have been substantially discredited."

The reputation of the Caucasus regions for longevity came about for several reasons:

- Old age is respected in the region, leading people to exaggerate their years.

- Anthropologists Trudy Turner of the University of Wisconsin and Mark Weiss of Wayne State University add, "The Soviet Union used these supposedly long-lived individuals for propaganda." Says Hayflick, "The resulting circus atmosphere tends to propel the age claims upward."

- Birth records and other trustworthy proof of long-ago birthdates are scarce. "There was really no convincing evidence that families in the Caucasus had produced several generations of centenarians," says Chopra. Georgakas adds, "The ferocious civil war of the 1990s has disrupted the orderly research . . . and may have destroyed vital records as well. . . . None of the Caucasus data can be accepted at face value."

But the people of the Caucasus may in fact live longer than people elsewhere—just not as long as some of the region's advocates have claimed. Georgakas notes that, according to a reputable expert on the region, "the rural Abkhazians did have unusual rates of longevity and reasonable health in old age."

Chopra mentions youthful rates of blood pressure among even the region's oldest citizens. And Ryback says that the Caucasians "[have] had less than one-tenth the number of strokes and about one-tenth the number of heart attacks as those living down in the plains. There was six times as much hypertension in the plains as in the mountains."

Why is this the case?

No one really knows, but Bellamy risks a guess: "It does appear as if . . . exceptionally long-lived survivors invariably [live] in small isolated communities where life-style and the social role of the elderly favor long life."

Until there is more research, though, the exact ages of the Caucasians and the life-lengthening powers of their way of life remain a matter of intrigue, fascination, and disagreement.

THE UNITED STATES

Which states in the United States will keep you alive the longest?

It's a matter of dispute, but Iowa and South Dakota seem the likeliest.

Iowa, says Chopra, has America's highest life expectancy, followed by South Dakota. While Hayflick puts Hawaii and Minnesota at the top of the list, he puts Iowa and South Dakota next.

"In general, the areas with the lowest rates [of death] were concentrated in the West Central and Mountain areas," Bellamy says. Iowa is in the center of the Central area—about half of it is on the western side—and South Dakota, which borders Iowa on the west, is split between the West Central and Mountain areas. (Minnesota, like Iowa, straddles the western and eastern sides of the Central area; it borders both Iowa and South Dakota.)

No one is completely sure why these states do so well in longevity.

WHICH STATES WILL KILL YOU FASTEST?

It's not clear.

"One of the first investigations in this direction demonstrated that in the United States, the highest rates [of death] from all causes occurred predominantly near the East Coast," Bellamy says.

On the other hand, according to government statistics, the state of Pennsylvania has a higher percentage of people over 65 than Utah and Alaska—which would seem to imply that people die older in Pennsylvania and that the state therefore has a *lower* death rate. But not necessarily. The birth rate in Utah and Alaska may run high, producing a high proportion of babies in the population and skewing the average age down. Or people over 65 may be moving out of Utah and Alaska, leaving mostly young people behind; perhaps people under 65 are getting out of Pennsylvania, leaving only older people behind.

So which states prevent you from living to a healthy old age? There simply isn't a confirmed definitive answer yet.

VILCABAMBA

In a village in Ecuador's Andes mountains, between the Peruvian border and the Pacific Ocean, sits Vilcabamba, which means "sacred valley." Vilcabamba has become famous for its long-lived people.

"Vilcabamba enjoys an association with good health dating back to the [time of the] Incas," writes Georgakas. Anthropologists Turner and Weiss report, "Captain George Coggeshall in 1825 . . . described several people who were more than 90 and 100 years old."

In more recent times, Vilcabamba's reputation for longevity has grown. "Popular interest was fanned by a spirited 1956 press conference in New York City featuring Javier Pereira, reputed to be 167, who had been brought to the United States by the owners of *Believe It or Not*, a syndicated newspaper feature," Georgakas says.

That was only the beginning. "In 1969 and 1970," Turner and Weiss report, "The government of Ecuador . . . sent Miguel Salvador, M.D., a cardiologist, to the area. . . . [He found] a high proportion of longevous individuals." In the early 1970s, gerontologist David Davies of London's University College met Vilcabamba's Miguel Carpio, who claimed to be 123, says Georgakas.

"A census taken in 1971 recorded nine individuals out of 819 [who] were over the age of 100. If this number is normalized, it would indicate 1,100 centenarians per 100,000 people"—as opposed to three per 100,000 in the United States—report Turner and Weiss.

Unfortunately, Walford says, "[further] investigations have failed to confirm [these reports]."

"Researchers found that ages above 70 were universally—and greatly—exaggerated," reports *Live Longer, Live Better*. Moore notes, "Investigators who visited Vilcabamba after a five-year absence discovered that the subjects claimed ages that were seven to ten years older than the previous visit."

Miguel Carpio was one of them. Georgakas reports that Carpio claimed to be 107 years old in 1970 but three years later said that he was 141.

Hayflick says, "In a study done in Vilcabamba in 1978, Richard B. Mazess (of the University of Wisconsin) and Sylvia H. Forman (of the University of Massachusetts) found that none of the . . . alleged centenarians investigated had, in fact, reached 100 years of age, and none of the . . . nonagenarians had reached 90."

Mazess and Forman's conclusion: "Individual longevity in Vilcabamba is little, if any, different from that found throughout the rest of the world." It seems there is, in fact, no valley of long life in the Andes.

HUNZA

The Hunza province in the Karakoram mountains of western Pakistan, near China and Afghanistan, is another of what *Live Longer, Live Better* calls "remote mountain Shangri-Las." Throughout the first three quarters of the twentieth century, travelers to the region reported meeting healthy, vigorous, and very old men and women. "According to their own testimony, the lives of the Hunzakuts . . . often stretch to a century or more," reports *Search for Immortality*.

But the reports couldn't be proven. "Some reported cases of healthy longevity . . . in the mountain valleys of Pakistan were improperly documented," says Willix. "The Hunzakuts, who have no written language, cannot even point to falsified birth certificates," adds Hayflick.

Moreover, *Search for Immortality* finds "some metaphorical snakes in this seeming paradise, including a high infant-mortality rate and disease-bearing parasites in [its] waters." Georgakas mentions vitamin and mineral deficiencies, malaria, dysentery, malnutrition, anemia, pneumonia, tuberculosis, and asthma in the region.

But, Georgakas goes on, there was a reason for the initial belief in the longevity of the Hunzakuts: "Most visitors had come to Hunza when the weather had cleared and the valley was in full bloom. By this time, many symptoms of malnutrition had been cured or ameliorated by the first harvest." So the Hunzakuts were apparently healthier at some times of the year than at others.

And so, in Georgakas's words, "Unless they are in the entourage of the Abominable Snowman, there are no supercentenarians in the Himalayas."

GEOGRAPHICAL FACTORS

Sometimes the actual place where you live doesn't matter as much as the *kind* of place that it is. Longevity can be stretched or cut short by the climate and the kind of community where you live.

CLIMATE

"Your cells are suited to particular environments," writes Michael Fossel in *Reversing Human Aging*. "The environment can be either too hot or too cold for cells to survive."

Or even too sunny. The elements of climate that the experts cite most often in connection with longevity are temperature and sunlight.

TEMPERATURE

Should you live in cold places or warm ones? Or does temperature matter at all?

Georgakas votes for cold. "Cooler climates [have] a slight advantage over warmer ones," he says. As an example, he offers the region of

Abkhazia, renowned for its long-lived residents. "[Its] mean temperature was 10 to 13 degrees Celsius [about 38 to 39 degrees Fahrenheit], with minimal seasonal variations."

But Case Western Reserve University's Cynthia Beall disagrees. "All causes of death (except cancers), and particularly deaths due to respiratory and arteriosclerotic disease, increase linearly with decreasing environmental temperatures from 20 degrees Celsius [about 43 degrees Fahrenheit] to −10 degrees Celsius [about 26 degrees Fahrenheit] in the United Kingdom and the United States." In other words, death rates rise as temperature drops.

Other experts toss out temperature altogether. Georgakas cites the work of the Russian Academy of Medical Science's Dimitri Chebotarev, who "eliminated climatic conditions as a major factor [in longevity]." Moore adds, "Long-lived nations can be found on tropical Caribbean islands and in the Arctic cold of Iceland and Finland."

How can these findings be reconciled with each other?

There's no answer. Perhaps it lies in Beall's observation that the data are incomplete. "All studies so far use samples from temperate-latitude industrial populations with high rates of cardiovascular disease and seasonal exposure to cold [like the United States] . . . Information from populations with low levels of cardiovascular disease or who are chronically exposed to unusual cold stress would be very useful"—but it isn't generally available yet.

Actual freezing to preserve life—cryonics—is another story, to be covered later in this book.

SUNLIGHT

Sunny places can be dangerous. If you live in California, Florida, or Texas, consider this:

- The American Cancer Society expects doctors to diagnose more than 500,000 new cases of skin cancer per year—and the sun will be responsible for most of them. "Ninety percent of all skin cancers are due to overexposure to the sun," Ford reports. The culprits are the sun's ultraviolet rays.

- Solar radiation weakens immunity. It hurts Langerhans cells, which "monitor substances throughout the epidermis to determine whether they are native to the body or foreign," says DiGiovanna. "When a Langerhans cell determines that a substance is foreign . . . it alters that substance so that other cells in the immune system can attack and eliminate it."

  But when intense sunlight repeatedly hits the body, it can damage Langerhans cells. "Exposing the body to intense sunlight for several hours can suppress immunity for up to 15 days," Ford explains.

- Even a so-called "healthy glow" can cause damage. "Tanning is the body's response to injury," Mindell explains. As Georgakas puts it, "Tanning is a defensive reaction of the body to the attack of the sun's ultraviolet rays, so consciously seeking a tan is to consciously age the skin prematurely."

What's more, you may not be able to undo sun damage. Ryback quotes UCLA dermatologist Tom Sternberg: "[Sun damage] is *cumulative, permanent,* and *progressive.*"

The bright side of the sun

"You could avoid skin damage by spending the rest of your life indoors, but that isn't a good idea," says Ford. After all, in *Aging: A Natural History*, professors Ricklefs and Finch call sunlight "necessary to our health."

Since ultraviolet rays create Vitamin D, which helps to keep bones strong, "people who are confined indoors for prolonged periods or who live at the extreme north or south latitudes will not get the sun exposure that is normal for their body chemistry," says Barnard. "Studies in Scandinavian countries," Georgakas adds, "indicate that one reason for that region's high rate of bone fractures may be that Scandinavians do not get enough exposure to sunlight during most of the year."

Clearly, you need to get some sun. But how much?

Your sunshine allotment

To absorb all the vitamin D that you need without courting skin cancer, most experts recommend about 10 minutes of sunlight per day.

But older people may need more time in the sun. "An older person must get more exposure to sunlight to produce the same amount of vitamin D [as a younger person]," DiGiovanna writes in *Human Aging*. "For optimal health, we should spend at least 30 minutes a day outdoors during daylight," says Ford.

Get in the sun when its rays are weakest and least likely to damage the skin. Most experts recommend avoiding the sun between 10 A.M. and 3 P.M.

Don't worry about missing a day. Once absorbed into the skin, vitamin D doesn't go away. "Vitamin D is then stored in fat and muscle, giving you a good supply for a rainy day or a whole string of rainy days," Barnard says.

Sunscreen and sunblock

If you're going to be in the sun for longer than 10 minutes, get a sunscreen or sunblock. When buying screens or blocks, look for SPF.

"The sun protection factor (SPF) is an index of degrees of protection in sunscreen against exposure to [ultraviolet] rays, ranging from 2 to 50," Ryback says. Barnard explains: "The SPF rating indicates the increase in the length of time it takes to burn. For example, if you would normally burn in 20 minutes under direct sun, a sunscreen with an SPF of 2 would protect you for 40 minutes, and one with an SPF of 10 would protect you for 200 minutes." Many experts recommend an SPF of at least 15, while some go as high as 30. In addition, Ford recommends using a sunscreen labeled "broad spectrum." Broad spectrum sunscreens protect against all kinds of ultraviolet rays (there are at least three), while other products may protect against fewer.

If you're in a sunny climate, apply sunscreen early—at least half an hour before going out into the sun, advise many authorities. According to *Age Erasers for Men*, "Applying sunscreen in the morning—every morning—could be your best defense," although this is a minority view.

Lay sunscreen on thick. "The SPFs are based on liberal applications," Ryback says.

Reapply sunscreen frequently (recommendations range from hourly to every two hours), especially if you're going to be in water. As Ryback says, "No sunscreen is completely waterproof." *Live Longer* adds, "Reapplication doesn't allow you to stay out longer; it simply restores the protection you had when you first put on sunscreen."

Finally, don't expect any sunscreen to be perfect.

- Mindell notes, "Although sunscreens can help prevent basal cell and squamous skin cancers, both of which are highly treatable if caught early, they do not protect against the more serious [cancer] melanoma."

- Sunscreens can't necessarily stop the rays that weaken immunity. Ryback adds, "Researchers at the M.D. Anderson Cancer Center in Houston report that even [strong] sunscreens can't prevent this effect."

- "Sunscreens and sunblocks may filter out the rays necessary to produce vitamin D," says Mindell.

- "Many people may be allergic to some of the ingredients used in sunscreens," Mindell says. "If in doubt, check with your physician."

Despite these problems, most experts recommend the use of sunscreens. But since no sunscreen is perfect, the experts also recommend other ways to combat the dangers of excessive sunlight.

Clothing

Georgakas notes that many long-lived people have enjoyed many years of working outdoors, which seems to contradict the prohibitions against spending too much time under the sun.

Perhaps those people evaded sun damage by wearing the proper clothes. "If you work outside during the summer months, I recommend wearing sun-protective clothing," Mindell says.

Not all clothes are created equal. "Wear clothes thick enough to block out the sun," Ford advises. "Cover the area with opaque clothing (denim is good)," *Live Longer, Live Better* recommends.

Thin clothes, by contrast, are weak clothes. Mindell says, "A summer-weight T-shirt offers protection equal to an SPF of 5 to 7 and only a 2 SPF when it is wet."

"Always wear a broad-brimmed hat," Ford advises. Mindell agrees: "It not only offers additional protection for your face but shields your scalp from the cancer-causing rays."

"Always wear appropriate sunglasses, too," *Live Longer, Live Better* recommends. "Your sunglasses should block virtually 100 percent of UV radiation. If you can see your eyes in a mirror with your sunglasses on, you don't have enough UV protection. Choose lenses large enough to prevent the sun from coming in on the sides, top, or bottom."

Medical cautions

Some diuretics, antibiotics, tranquilizers, and antihistamines can increase sensitivity to sunlight, causing skin damage. Mindell says, "If you're taking any medication, be sure to check with your physician before spending time outdoors."

Tanning without sun

If you yearn for a tan, many experts recommend various dyes, ointments, and creams. "New cosmetic products do the job safely and temporarily without the sun by dyeing the outermost cells," Barnard says. "In a few days, your tanned cells are sloughed off, and normal skin color returns."

RURAL VERSUS URBAN

Country folks have it all over city slickers. "Rural farm areas have the lowest statistical death rates from all causes," Bellamy reports.

What advantages do rural areas have? The evidence isn't conclusive, except for one fact—rural areas aren't urban ones. As Chopra says, "A city is essentially a monolithic stress machine, cranking out noise and air pollution, along with excessive speed, overcrowding, crime, and rudeness."

Among the best nonurban places may be the high ones. "Living in the mountains, specifically at heights of between 5,000 and 10,000 feet, may well have a salubrious effect on aging persons," *Search for Immortality* says. Bellamy adds, "Deaths from cardiovascular and renal disease [are] linked with regions of high rainfall and low elevation."

While rural areas at high elevations may have advantages, there are always exceptions. Moore notes that people live long "packed densely together in the metropolitan confines of Hong Kong, and scattered thinly across the vast expanses of Canada and Australia."

In other words, rural places are good—but they're not the only life-stretching places to live, nor is rural life the most important factor in longevity.

POLLUTED PLACES

No shocker here: Pollution can shorten life.

"Wherever there is a concentration of petrochemical industries, there is a cancer hot spot," Georgakas says. For example, says Barnard, "Women who live near toxic waste sites do in fact have higher rates of breast cancer."

"The most prominent example is the infamous cancer alley of New Jersey, which coincides with the industrial complex bordering the New Jersey Turnpike," says Georgakas. "Communities on Staten Island and in Brooklyn, separated from the source of contamination by miles of water, are also affected because of the prevailing westerly winds."

One pollution problem that longevity experts often mention is water. Be careful about where you get your water, advises Georgakas. Dumping of pollutants, he says, "occurs in every American waterway. . . . From the Hudson to the Columbia, the story is the same: the mighty rivers of America have become so severely polluted that the purification systems of many cities are no longer adequate to deal with the problem."

And, Georgakas says, "People who live in the country or in small towns are not necessarily exempt from these water-pollution wells."

If you're in doubt as to your region's water safety, he concludes, "assistance is available from the Environmental Protection Agency and local public-health officers. If the water proves to be less than satisfactory, one should use bottled water provided by a responsible company. If one is considering a filtration device for faucets, it is best to check with a good consumer guide."

SMOKING

SIMPLY PUT, SMOKING KILLS.

- Chopra mentions a UCLA study of life-style choices that led to early death: "At the top of the list for those who died earliest in the study were sedentary life-style and smoking."

- The World Health Organization reports that smokers have higher death rates than nonsmokers. And the death rate rises with the more cigarettes that a person smokes in a day, the more years that he's smoked, and the younger he was when he started smoking.

- Moore describes a study in which "the mortality rate among those who smoked a pack a day was more than twice as high as among those who had never smoked." In another study, "among women who reached age 25, . . . 45 percent of heavy smokers died before age 70, compared with only 15 percent of nonsmokers."

- "If it doesn't kill you—and one in five people worldwide die from smoking-related diseases every year—it will most certainly take years off your life," the *Age Erasers* books declare. According to Moore's mortality-rate study, "among those 35 to 45 years old, [smoking] reduced life expectancy by seven years."

- "No one who continues to smoke can hope to retard or reverse the aging process," Ford says. Says University of California at San Francisco professor Margaret Chesney, "If you want to radically slow down the aging process and live longer, stop smoking."

SMOKING: THE EFFECTS

What exactly does smoking do?

Dr. Douglas Jorenby of the University of Wisconsin at Madison's Center for Tobacco Research and Intervention says, "The effects of smoking are distributed so much throughout the entire body that it has an impact on virtually any diseases you can think of."

HEART DISEASE

Smoking damages the heart.

- The American Heart Association says that almost one-fifth of heart-disease deaths result from cigarette smoking. The Heart Association adds that blood clots, which contribute to the great majority of heart attacks, are often caused by smoking. A British Medical Association survey reveals that heavy smokers have 15 times the risk of dying by heart attack before age 45 than non-smokers do.

- "Up to 40 percent of CAD [coronary artery disease] deaths each year are believed to be due to smoke-related problems," says Mindell.

- When it comes to developing atherosclerosis, says DiGiovanna, "Smoking almost doubles the risk."

- According to the *Age Erasers* books, "Smoking . . . puts you at increased risk for stroke by speeding up clogging in the carotid arteries." As a result, Mindell says, "If you smoke, you are twice as likely to have a stroke than a nonsmoker."

CANCER

Smoking is infamous for its connection to cancer.

- A United Nations World Health Organization report published in 1997 blamed smoking for nearly 15 percent of all cancers.

- "The major contributing causes to the top three cancer killers for women (breast cancer, colonic cancer, and lung cancer) and the two for men (lung cancer and colonic cancer) are tobacco smoking and fat-laden diets," Georgakas explains.

- "Smokers are three times more likely to die of cancer than nonsmokers," says *Live Longer, Live Better.* In particular, "smokers are ten times more likely to develop lung cancer [than nonsmokers]," the *Age Erasers* books report.

OTHER LUNG DISEASES

"Of all the factors that influence lung function, smoking continues to produce the greatest amount of disability," says the American Geriatrics Society. "Smoking is the primary cause in the overwhelming majority of people with COPD [chronic obstructive pulmonary disease]." COPDs include emphysema, chronic bronchitis, and asthma.

OTHER EFFECTS

Smoking hurts in many other ways.

- In *18 Natural Ways,* Ford writes, "Cigarette smoking is the most potent promoter of free radicals in existence." Not only does it encourage the body to create free radicals, but, says Moore, "Cigarette smoke is [itself] rich in free radicals."

- The University of Wisconsin's Jorenby says "Even if smoking is not a causal factor in a particular disease, it can certainly exacerbate it. For instance, we know that smoking doesn't cause diabetes, but people with diabetes who smoke have a much worse prognosis than those who don't."

- And, smoking can affect the mind and emotions. Indiana University sociologist Richard Jenks says, "Smokers tend to feel they have less control over their lives, and feel less satisfied with their lives, than nonsmokers."

SMOKING: THE DEFENSE

It's tough to stop smoking. If you smoke, you may refuse to stop because of one, some, or all of the following reasons:

THE SLIMNESS DEFENSE

A lean body is likely to live a long time, and "smokers are often leaner than nonsmokers," says Barnard.

Why does this happen? "Nicotine slightly curbs the appetite," explains *Age Erasers for Women.* Moreover, cigarettes increase noradrenaline, a hormone that aids the body in dropping pounds.

But, Barnard says, "you don't need to smoke to get that slimming effect. It comes to you in a very healthy way, as part of a carbohydrate-rich diet," since carbohydrates are in fat and can help the body step up noradrenaline production.

If you quit smoking, you may gain weight—many ex-smokers gain five to eight pounds—but "those few extra pounds are not nearly the danger to your health that smoking is," *Live Longer* declares. Besides, "any weight gain will be temporary," Ryback says.

THE RELAXATION DEFENSE

Some people claim that smoking can relax you, thereby fighting stress. To that claim, Georgakas says, "The illusionary relief offered by narcotics, alcohol, or tobacco is counterproductive, speeding up rather than retarding premature aging."

So tobacco may help you feel better temporarily, but it's aging you over the long run.

THE "SMOG IS WORSE" DEFENSE

Smoking, it's been said, is no worse than living in a big city with its attendant smog. Georgakas disputes that contention, calling tobacco smoke "far more dangerous than air pollution."

He explains, "This error is based on misinterpretation of studies such as the one [that] found that a person standing in Manhattan's Herald Square for 24 hours would be exposed to the same amount of pollutants as [is] found in two packs of cigarettes."

Georgakas notes that Herald Square is more polluted than most urban spots; no one would stand there for 24 hours; Herald Square's pollutants get dispersed into the air, while tobacco smoke stays concentrated within the body; and tobacco smoke is inhaled from the mouth straight into the lungs, whereas most people breathe air through the nose, which can filter out some of the pollutants.

So tobacco smoke is worse than smog.

THE GEEZER DEFENSE

Everyone's heard of how George Burns smoked cigars into old age. And he hasn't been the only one to do so.

So is smoking one way to live long?

No. Those smokers who live a long time are the exceptions. Some people will smoke and age quite well because smoking isn't a sure killer; but it's a big risk factor.

A comparison: Driving recklessly isn't a sure killer. But it raises the risk of death by car crash. Just as some people can drive at wild speeds every day and never get a scratch, other people can smoke a pack a day and live to be 100.

But that's not the way to bet.

THE ANTIOXIDANT DEFENSE

This defense is based on the idea that some substances can overcome the damage caused by smoking. "If you choose to drink or smoke, you can mitigate their effects by taking antioxidants and by exercising and eating right," Willix says.

Mitigate the effects, yes. Eliminate them, no.

Georgakas points out that smoking can hurt even someone who eats right, exercises, and keeps a positive, relaxed attitude: "Smoking is so deadly it undermines all benefits from an otherwise longevous life-style." Willix agrees: "There's no course of antioxidant therapy or treatment I know of that will remove completely (or even to a significant degree) the effects of smoking and drinking."

"I'M ALREADY DOOMED, SO I MAY AS WELL KEEP SMOKING."

People use this fatalistic approach as an excuse. But it doesn't work. "It's never too late to quit," Ryback says.

Some proof:

- "If you're an otherwise healthy 35-year-old who stops smoking, you'll add about seven years to your life," Willix declares. "If you quit before age 40, you can add five years to your life. If you quit by age 50, you can add three years," Ryback says.

- *Live Longer, Live Better* reports, "Quitting smoking after the age of 50 cuts your risk of heart disease in half, leads to a better outcome if you already have a smoking-related disease, and reduces your number of headaches, stomachaches, and respiratory infections."

- "If you've been smoking up to the age of 70 and quit then, you can still benefit by one additional year of life," Ryback says.

You can erase some effects of smoking completely. *Live Longer, Live Better* says, "No matter what your age, not smoking for 15 years makes your health risks comparable to those of people who never smoked." Ryback adds, "As long as cancer has not yet started, the effects of smoking are definitely reversible."

For instance:

- Says *Age Erasers for Women*, "The risk of stroke dropped to normal levels for women two to four years after they quit."

- *Living Well* says, "The senior who stops cigarette smoking returns to an average risk of heart attack after only two years and a nearly normal risk of lung cancer after ten."

- The *Age Erasers* books note, "Just one year after you quit smoking, your risk for heart disease is cut in half, and after three years, your risk becomes comparable to that of someone who never touched a cigarette."

"IN THAT CASE, I DON'T HAVE TO STOP NOW. I CAN QUIT ANYTIME AND REGAIN MY HEALTH."

Not exactly. While some body systems can return to normal, many others can't. "The development of emphysema is arrested [in] many people when they stop smoking, although this condition does not reverse," Fries says.

The later you quit smoking, the more damage your body will have sustained, and the longer it will take to recover.

QUITTING

The first step is mental. "Half the trouble with quitting smoking," Ryback says, "is overcoming the denial that smoking is a form of systematic suicide."

Once you accept the dangers of smoking and the need to quit, "decide firmly that you really want to do it," Fries advises. "If you have not made a clear decision to quit, then . . . you will not be successful, no matter what techniques you use," Ryback says.

There are various techniques for quitting smoking:

THE QUIT DATE

Pick a date for your last cigarette. This is a good way to prepare yourself to stop smoking.

The quit date should be about two to four weeks in the future. "A date two to four weeks away is close enough to take seriously, but [it] also allows you time to get prepared," says *Live Longer, Live Better*.

To get ready for the quit date:

- Cut down. *Live Longer* recommends letting yourself smoke in only one room. Fries suggests: "Only keep in the cigarette pack those cigarettes you are going to allow yourself that day. Smoke the cigarettes only halfway down before extinguishing them."

- Deflect the urges. When you feel the need to smoke, exercise or drink juice instead, *Live Longer* suggests. Says Don Powell, Ph.D., of the American Institute for Preventive Medicine: "Hold off lighting up for five minutes. . . . After another few days, extend it to 15 minutes, and so on."

- Get support. Suggests *Live Longer*, "After you pick a date to quit, let friends and family members know so that they can help you." They can give you encouragement and help you stay away from situations in which you're likely to smoke.

ON THE QUIT DAY

Ready? Begin.

- Remove all cigarettes and other smoking paraphernalia from work and home.

- Write down the times and situations when you smoke. At those times, do something else.

  A commonly suggested example of "something else" is exercise. "Exercise will take your mind off the smoking change, and it will decrease the tendency to gain weight in the early weeks after stopping smoking," Fries says. *Staying Young* agrees: "The high you get from natural 'feel good' chemicals released by exercise will replace the stimulating lift you may be accustomed to getting from nicotine."

- Get help. "Although quitting cold turkey is the most popular method [of quitting], it is also the least successful, having a success rate of only 5 percent," the *Age Erasers* books report.

  If you are not in that small percentage, visit a medical doctor or psychologist, or join a smoking-cessation program. "Smoking-cessation programs often include counseling, relaxation training, hypnosis, or some other form of behavioral therapy," explains *Staying Young*.

  To find a program, call the American Cancer Society, the American Heart Association, or the American Lung Association.

WITHDRAWAL SYMPTOMS

Nicotine is addictive. Withdrawal can make you irritable or nervous; it can give you headaches, gastrointestinal problems, or coughing fits; it can make you sleepless or drowsy.

Withdrawal can last from two days to three months, with the first days being the hardest. To fight the symptoms:

- Soothe yourself. Many experts recommend meditation and relaxation to help you through the rough times of quitting.

- Drink fruit juice, particularly orange juice. The *Age Erasers* books explain, "OJ makes your urine more acidic, which clears nicotine from your body faster, says Thomas Cooper, D.D.S., a nicotine dependency researcher."

- Talk to yourself. "Label urges and irritability as signs of success, as reminders that you've conquered smoking," says Ryback. "Imagine it's the flu," suggest the *Age Erasers* books, which quote Dr. Jorenby: "A lot of withdrawal symptoms are similar to the flu. . . . But you will get over it."

- Try nicotine patches or nicotine gum. Both are available by prescription. "Since they dispense some nicotine to your system, they eliminate many of the physical symptoms of nicotine withdrawal," Willix explains.

  But be careful with gum and patches. Since, like cigarettes, they pour nicotine into the body, most experts recommend using them for only a few months.

RELAPSES

If you fall back into smoking, don't worry. Just try again. "It takes most smokers three or four unsuccessful attempts before they give up cigarettes for good," reports *Live Longer*.

The encouraging news is that those people do in fact give up smoking—permanently. "For [the ones] who persist," says Ryback, "success is virtually guaranteed."

SMOKING AT SECOND HAND

Tobacco companies may argue this one until their last gasp, but second-hand smoke is a killer.

Live Longer, Live Better explains, "[Smoking] fills the room with carbon monoxide emissions, benzene, ammonia, nicotine, and carcinogenic tars." Says Georgakas: "Any small room with even one person smoking in it will have a higher level of carbon monoxide, carcinogens, and toxins than the entrance to most factories. The dangers to longevity are acute."

Among those dangers:

- *Live Longer* reports, "The nonsmoking spouses of smokers face a 30 percent higher risk of dying of lung cancer than those who have nonsmoking partners." The *Age Erasers* books say, "Up to 8,000 lung cancer deaths a year among nonsmokers can be attributed to secondhand smoke."

- A decade-long study conducted at Harvard University followed more than 30,000 nonsmoking women. The results, published by the medical journal *Circulation* in 1997, found that the women who regularly breathed secondhand smoke suffered nearly double the risk of heart disease as the women who didn't inhale smoke.

To preserve your longevity, stay away from smoke—and ask smokers to put their lights out.

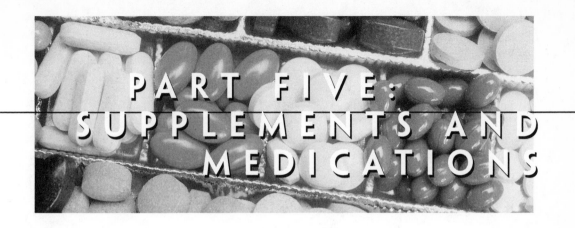

PART FIVE:
SUPPLEMENTS AND
MEDICATIONS

IN THE BABYLONIAN EPIC OF GILGAMESH, WRITES CAROL ORLOCK IN *The End of Aging,* the hero "heads out looking for the plant of eternal youth, supposedly located at the bottom of the sea." And he finds it. But, writes Georgakas in *The Methuselah Factors,* "before he could benefit from its rejuvenating powers, it was stolen from him by a serpent seeking a new skin."

And so has gone the search for a medication, formula, or procedure to extend life and health. The elixir often disappears when it looks most promising.

ANCIENT DAYS

In *How and Why We Age,* Hayflick describes an Egyptian papyrus dating back at least 3,500 years, which mentions an ointment that allegedly turns an old man into a youth of 20. In the myths of ancient Greece, says Orlock, Jason the Argonaut gathered "pebbles from the Orient, hoarfrost gathered by moonlight, parts from a horned owl, the entrails of a were-wolf, and the head of a 900-year-old crow" into a potion that "turned back the clock 40 years."

The Roman poet Ovid, in his *Metamorphoses,* introduced the idea of injecting life-sustaining substances directly into the veins—specifically the veins of the Greek king Aeson. "After brewing up ram's blood, owl's flesh, snakeskin, and a variety of roots, herbs, and plants, [the sorceress] Medea plunged her dagger into a vein in the old man's throat and poured in the magic mixture; the king leaped form his sickbed, filled with strength he had not felt for 40 years," reports *Search for Immortality.*

Over the next several centuries, doctors and frauds alike have pro-moted alchemy, blood transfusions, and hormones and sexual organs from various sources (monkey glands, for example) as hopes for long life.

BOGOMOLETZ'S SERUM

In the 1940s, Ukrainian scientist Alexander Bogomoletz, director of the Kiev Institute of Experimental Biology and Pathology, announced to wide public attention the creation of antireticular cytotoxic serum. He injected this vaccine into whole animal cells with the goal of producing exceptionally powerful antibodies in the recipient.

Unfortunately, says Hayflick, "there is no evidence that antibodies produced by inoculating whole animal cells are beneficial. In fact, there is the real threat that antibodies . . . will attack [the] cells in a human recipient, causing severe reaction and perhaps death."

By the end of the decade, says Georgakas, "[Bogomoletz's] claim was withdrawn."

GEROVITAL

"In the mid-1950s, a new combination called Gerovital, which had been devised by Dr. Ana Aslan of Rumania, was thought capable of revitalizing the body," says Georgakas. Hayflick reports, "Believers from Western countries made sales skyrocket. With the proceeds, she built a large research institute and earned substantial amounts of hard foreign currency."

Although Aslan is now dead, "a health cult has emerged around Aslan's work. In major American cities, Gerovital is still sold clandestinely as a 'forbidden' youth drug," says Georgakas.

Don't buy it. Gerovital doesn't work. Studies in the United States, United Kingdom, and Soviet Union have proved it worthless.

What is Gerovital? Some benzoic acid, some potassium metabisulfate, and, according to Georgakas, mostly procaine hydrochloride—alias Novocain.

AND TODAY

According to *Aging on Hold*: "Herbal brews, organ extracts, bubbling elixirs—such magic potions to restore lost youth have long been the stuff of dreams. But now that real science has joined the pursuit with its own exotic blends—hormones, steroids, and growth factors—some of the dreams are within reach.

"Emboldened by recent breakthroughs in understanding the aging process, researchers are testing chemicals with the potential to reset biological clocks and enable men and women to retard the rigors of time."

Not all of the potions are safe or effective, though. Hayflick explains: "The monkey-gland injections of several decades ago have given way to the life-extension movement, whose proponents distribute a formidable array of chemicals through mail-order houses, health-food stores, and youth doctors. Because they are sold as dietary supplements, with no therapeutic claims on the label, they escape supervision by the Food and Drug Administration."

The following sections will examine these substances.

DIETARY SUPPLEMENTS

DIETARY SUPPLEMENTS—USUALLY PILLS CONTAINING VITAMINS, minerals, hormones, or other substances—are among the most controversial substances involving longevity. Entire books promote or denounce them. It's only fair to give both sides of the argument.

THE POSITIVE SIDE

Some reasons for supplements:

- Scientific studies support them. Dr. Richard Deeb writes in *Live to Be 100+*: "In many animal studies, supplementation with antioxidants has yielded beneficial results. Supplementation also seems to have positive effects on humans. Based on the results of such studies, it appears prudent to supplement one's diet with additional antioxidants."

- They may help people overcome the unhealthy assaults of modern life. "We are exposed to increased barrages from our polluted environment," writes Jean Carper in *Stop Aging Now!* "We require heroic countermeasures in the form of antioxidant vitamins and minerals."

- We may need them to live longer than nature intended. Carper mentions the view of Denham Harman, who first theorized about free radicals and antioxidants: "Nature's intent is to dump us after middle age when we have completed our procreation duties. To survive longer in good health, he says, we need the extra boost from antioxidants"—including antioxidant supplements.

- We need to fill in the gaps in our diets. In *18 Natural Ways to Look and Feel Half Your Age,* Norman Ford says, "Even when eating a nutritious diet, four out of every five Americans over age 50 do not get the full range of vitamins and minerals they need from their food." Neil Barnard explains in *Eat Right, Live Longer,* "Those who center their diets on meat and dairy products are likely to miss out on a broad range of antioxidants." Consequently, writes Stanford's Walter Bortz in *Dare to Be 100,* "I often prescribe vitamins to older patients, particularly if I feel they are at risk for not eating the traditional well-balanced menu."

- Even a good diet may not have enough nutrients. Carper says, "Certain key vitamins in doses exceeding those in food promise protection against aging and disease far beyond all previous expectations."

The *Age Erasers* books conclude: "More research is being conducted to determine the exact form and amount of the antioxidants needed for optimal health and disease protection. Until then, most researchers believe we can best protect ourselves with a combination of diet and supplements."

THE NEGATIVE SIDE

And now, some responsible opposing viewpoints:

- The evidence for supplements is not conclusive. *Search for Immortality* reports, "The claims made for diet supplements leave most mainstream scientists cold." George Washington University's Moore, examining studies on antioxidant supplements, finds no record of success in humans "and a mixture of failure and success in animal experiments." Orlock says, "Studies testing supplements often provide insignificant or negative results."

- Supplements are narrow in scope. *Dr. Bob Arnot's Guide to Turning Back the Clock* cites the work of Harvard Medical School's Charles Hennekens, M.D.: "The extraction process [involved in making supplements] leaves behind hundreds of different components of real food, the most critical of which are called phytochemicals, key disease-fighting chemicals." Says Ford, "No [supplement] can supply the bonanza of antioxidants, phytochemicals, and fiber found in foods that grow on plants."

- Antioxidants in high doses may weaken each other's effects. As Barnard notes, "Beta carotene supplements can reduce the amount of vitamin E in the blood by as much as 40 percent."

- The body itself may weaken the supplements. In *Ageless Body, Timeless Mind*, Chopra explains, "Many [supplements] would be nullified by digestive juices in the mouth, stomach, and intestines long before they got to the cells they were meant to protect."

SO WHAT SHOULD YOU DO?

Since supplements are a matter of controversy—as Orlock says, "The evidence is accumulating rapidly, but the jury is still very much out"—caution is probably sensible.

For one thing, try a healthy diet before you try supplements. Nutritionist Jeffrey Blumberg of Tufts University's Human Nutrition Research Center notes, "[Supplements] are not 'magic bullets' and work best in conjunction with healthy nutritional practices . . . such as eating low-fat, high-fiber meals." Or as UCLA's Walford puts it in *The Anti-Aging Plan*, "Untrimmed hamburger on white bread, topped off with a candy bar and a handful of pills, will not suffice."

Second, if you want to try supplements, check with your doctor before dosing yourself.

Since supplements may be beneficial—and since, beneficial or not, many people take them—the following sections will cover them in detail.

RDAS

Before discussing individual supplements, a note on nomenclature. The makers of supplements often refer to RDAs, but they don't always bother to explain them.

WHAT ARE THE RDAS?

"The U.S. Recommended Daily Allowances, or RDAs," explains Orlock, "[were] developed to monitor the nutritional needs of military recruits during World War II. . . . These measures were later revised downward somewhat, more in line with the nutritional needs of adult women."

RDAs can be confusing because they come in two types. The Recommended *Dietary* Allowances come from the Food and Nutrition Board of the National Academy of Sciences, says DiGiovanna in *Human Aging*. "[These] RDAs provide enough of each nutrient to maintain good health and are higher than the amounts needed just to survive." DiGiovanna notes that these RDAs vary according to a person's weight, height, age, and gender.

Then there are the Recommended *Daily* Allowances. "To assist consumers and those evaluating and planning diets, the Food and Drug Administration used the values in the RDAs to develop the U.S. Recommended Daily Allowance (U.S. RDA) for many nutrients," says DiGiovanna. "The labels on many packaged foods list the percentages of the U.S. RDA for many nutrients."

Generally speaking, most people who refer to RDAs probably mean U.S. RDAs.

SPECIFIC SUPPLEMENTS: VITAMINS

Of all the supplements, vitamin pills are probably the most common and the most popular. But some vitamins carry more benefits—and dangers—than others.

VITAMIN A AND BETA CAROTENE

Vitamin A

Vitamin A can fight cancer. But vitamin A supplements may be another story. "For every study that shows benefits [of vitamin A supplements]," says Bortz, "there is another study that doesn't."

- Carper notes that half the people over 60 need supplements because they don't get enough vitamin A. Yet the University of

Arizona's William Stini says, "Elderly individuals often exhibit elevated [blood] serum levels of vitamin A"—in other words, too much vitamin A.

- Vitamin A seems to fight one kind of cancer yet promote another kind. A Johns Hopkins University study from 1994 found that vitamins A, C, and E did cut the risk of basal cell carcinoma, a common cancer, by 70 percent. But as *Live Longer, Live Better* observes, "At least one long-term study found that men who took vitamin A supplements actually had a somewhat higher incidence of lung cancer than those who did not."

- Kedar Prasad, Ph.D., of the Center for Vitamins and Cancer Research at the University of Colorado recommends 5,000 to 10,000 IU (international units) of vitamin A daily, while other experts warn that amounts in that range or higher "can produce fatigue and weakness, cause liver dysfunction [and] headache, produce high calcium in the blood, and reduce the number of circulating white blood cells" (according to the American Geriatrics Society).

No wonder experts such as Ranjit Chandra (of the Memorial University of Newfoundland in St. John's and the World Health Organization Center of Nutritional Immunology) recommend avoiding vitamin A supplements.

A better way to get vitamin A, according to several experts, is to take supplements of its relative, beta carotene.

Beta carotene

These supplements have multiple powers.

- Beta carotene supplements may be able to fight cancer. Pacific Western University's Earl Mindell, in *Earl Mindell's Anti-Aging Bible,* mentions a study in which "people with oral lesions were given 60 milligrams (100,000 international units) of beta carotene daily. After six months, most of the patients experienced a 50 percent reduction or more in the number of mouth lesions, thus reducing their risk of developing oral cancers."

What's more, the U.S. National Cancer Institute studied a group of Chinese who ingested beta carotene (as well as vitamin E and selenium). In 1993, the institute announced its findings: their rate of death by cancer dropped by 13 percent in five years.

• Beta carotene supplements can fight heart disease and stroke. "Among a group of 300 men at high risk for heart disease, consuming extra beta carotene was linked to a 50 percent reduction in the likelihood of heart attack and stroke," Orlock explains. Carper says, "A Harvard study showed that male physicians who took 50-milligram supplements of beta carotene . . . had only half as many fatal heart attacks, strokes, and heart disease incidents in general as doctors taking a dummy pill."

• And, Carper says, "Beta carotene supplements can greatly improve the makeup of your immune cells, according to tests at the University of Arizona."

On the other hand, a Finnish study of 29,000 smokers concluded that "beta carotene supplementation . . . might actually contribute to cancer," says Orlock. As a result, Carper says, "Most researchers now warn current smokers against taking single high doses of beta carotene supplements."

If you don't smoke, the experts who recommend beta carotene say that you should take from 6 to 30 milligrams per day, with most experts recommending 15 milligrams.

How much is too much? "It is almost impossible to consume toxic levels of beta carotene," say the *Age Erasers* books, based on the testimony of Dr. Jeffrey Blumberg of Tufts University. Says Mindell, "In fact, many studies used dosages as high as 50 milligrams of beta carotene without any problem."

There is one drawback to excessively high doses of beta carotene. They can turn the skin orange or yellow.

Fortunately, cutting back will eliminate that effect.

THE B VITAMINS

Vitamin B₃ (niacin)

Niacin can lower cholesterol. In fact, Ryback reports in *Look Ten Years Younger, Live Ten Years Longer,* "Niacin has the best track record for safety of all cholesterol-lowering drugs and is the least expensive by far."

Vegetarians may have a special need for niacin supplements. Except for enriched-grain and whole-grain breads, plant products contain little niacin. So supplements may be the vegetarian's only choice.

But supplements can be harmful. Mindell says, "High doses of niacin can be toxic to your liver." *Staying Young* reports that niacin may also hurt kidneys. (Diabetics are especially susceptible to niacin's negative effects.)

Before taking any supplement, it's good to see a doctor. That advice applies doubly to niacin.

Vitamin B₆ (pyridoxine)

Vitamin B₆ supplements can help to fight cancer, says Carper. She adds that they can also control levels of homocysteine, an amino acid. *Staying Young* reports, "A study by Paul F. Jacques, Sc.D., assistant professor at the school of Nutrition at Tufts University—U.S. Department of Agriculture Human Nutrition Research Center on Aging, Boston, suggests that high homocysteine levels might explain heart attacks in people with no apparent risk factors."

Although B₆ supplements appear harmless when taken in moderate doses, not everyone favors them. "One can make an arguable case for [B₆ supplements]," admits Walford, "but the evidence is marginal as to long-term benefits." Besides, he says, you don't need B₆ supplements, "assuming you are eating a balanced mixture of wholesome foods."

The authorities who do recommend B₆ supplements suggest 50 to 100 milligrams per day, especially for men with prostate trouble or women who are suffering from moodiness or depression due to menopause.

But don't overdose. Daily doses over 200 milligrams can damage the nervous system.

Vitamin B₁₂ (cobalamin)

If you don't have enough B_{12} in your body, Chopra says, you can suffer symptoms of senility. Fortunately, Carper observes, "taking vitamin B_{12} pills usually prevents this mental deterioration."

Vegetarians over age 60 are prime candidates for B_{12} supplements, the experts say. B_{12} comes from animal products, not plant-based foods (except for enriched breakfast cereals), so vegetarians can become deficient in it; many older people have atrophic gastritis, a condition that makes it harder for them to absorb B_{12} from food.

Carper recommends 500 to 1,000 micrograms. But larger doses may be safe as well. To repeat the usual advice: check with your doctor before dosing yourself.

Folic acid (also called folate or folacin)

This B vitamin can fight heart disease, cancer, and depression, and help the body stay immune to disease. Unfortunately, "the average American over 50 is woefully deficient in folic acid," Carper says. For such people, the experts recommend doses of 400 to 1,000 micrograms per day.

Higher doses—particularly those edging close to 10,000 micrograms or more— "could mask symptoms of B_{12} deficiency and pernicious anemia," Carper says. "If you have any reason to suspect you might have this condition, check it out before taking over 1,000 micrograms of folic acid a day."

Other B vitamins

Vitamins B_1 (thiamine) and B_2 (riboflavin) don't get as much mention in the literature on supplements as their fellow Bs do. The experts simply don't spend as much time touting or refuting their powers. Check with a doctor before taking them.

VITAMIN C

Vitamin C supplements are controversial. While Ford says, "It is entirely possible to obtain sufficient vitamin C from a diet high in fresh fruits and vegetables," he adds that getting that much isn't easy— "Unless you eat at least five servings of fresh fruit per day, you may benefit from a vitamin C supplement." Moreover, Carper quotes University of Alabama emeritus professor Emanual Cheraskin, who says, "Virtually nobody gets enough vitamin C"; Carper believes that almost nobody can do without vitamin C supplements.

What supplements can do

Vitamin C supplements can keep the body alive in many ways:

- "One decade-long study of 11,348 adults concluded that men who took 300 milligrams per day of supplemental vitamin C had a mortality rate 41 percent lower than men who took only 50 milligrams," Ford says.

- Vitamin C can lower the risk of heart disease. "The U.S. government's First National Health and Nutrition Examination Survey found that Americans who regularly took vitamin C supplements had 37 percent fewer heart attacks [than people who didn't]," says Carper. She quotes UCLA researcher James Enstrom: "A 35-year-old man who eats vitamin C-rich foods and takes vitamin C supplements will slash his chances of heart disease death by two-thirds and live 6.3 years longer."

- According to Kedar Prasad, Ph.D., of the Center for Vitamins and Cancer Research, vitamin C supplements strengthen your body's immune system. The National Cancer Institute testifies that vitamin C in doses available only in supplements—5,000 to 10,000 milligrams a day—raises immunity against disease.

- Vitamin C, according to Prasad, may help to fight cancer by strengthening the immune system to the point where it "can destroy newly formed cancer cells before they multiply."

In experiments on rats, "large doses of vitamin C reduce the number of rats developing colon cancer in response to a chemical carcinogen," Barnard says. "And vitamin C reduces the incidence of abnormalities in the DNA (the genetic material, abnormalities of which are often associated with later cancer development) of human workers exposed to coal tar products."

Dosage

Most experts recommend 500 to 1,000 milligrams per day, with many leaning toward the higher end of that range.

Going beyond 1,000 milligrams seems unnecessary. Ford says, "Since 250 to 500 milligrams of vitamin C will completely saturate every cell in the body, taking megadoses of this vitamin seems of dubious benefit. Instead, most nutritionists recommend taking a maximum of one gram [1,000 milligrams] daily, preferably in the form of two 250- to 500-milligram supplements taken twelve hours apart." Carper adds, "Throwing down a couple of 500-milligram pills at one time, particularly in the morning, instead of taking them throughout the day, cheats your cells because much of it is excreted in your urine."

Cautions

Nobel Prize winner Linus Pauling, perhaps the twentieth century's strongest advocate of vitamin C, recommended up to 12,000 milligrams a day, and he lived to age 93. But Pauling "stressed very strongly that each individual has a unique biochemistry that calls for different amounts of vitamin C, ranging from as little as one-quarter of a gram [250 milligrams] to 20 or more grams [20,000 or more milligrams] per day," Ryback explains.

There are two well-known consequences of consuming too much vitamin C.

- *The American Geriatrics Society's Complete Guide to Aging & Health* says, "Megadoses of vitamin C can produce kidney stones."

Not everyone believes this claim. According to Barnard, Pauling believed there was no proof that vitamin C causes kidney stones. And Cornell University's Linda Gerber and Ohio State University's Douglas Crews write in *Biological Anthropology*, "Formation of oxalate stones in the kidney has been suggested as an example of a condition related to excessive vitamin C intake; however, recent data do not support this association."

So the kidney stone-vitamin C connection may be a chimera.

"Vitamin C [has a] tendency to increase iron absorption," Barnard says. If the body absorbs too much iron, free radical damage, cancer, diabetes, and heart disease can result.

Carper finds that excess vitamin C is likeliest to cause excess iron absorption in people who have "genetic disorders in handling iron, notably a condition called hemochromatosis. Such persons should consult a physician before taking vitamin C supplements."

Of course, consulting a physician before dosing oneself is a good idea in any case.

VITAMIN D

Vitamin D can help to keep bones strong and fight off osteoporosis. Carper says, "Vitamin D supplements after a year can dramatically prevent broken bones even in 80-year-olds."

Who needs vitamin D? Vegetarians (vitamin D comes from eggs, fish, and milk) or people who don't get much sun. People with brittle or weak bones—especially older people—may benefit, too.

According to the experts, most people who need more vitamin D can do well on a supplement of 200 IU (five micrograms) per day. People with an especially strong need—such as older people who don't get their vitamin D through sunlight or diet—may require 600 IU. But too much—even as little as 400 IU, says Barnard—is "potentially toxic and should be avoided."

In fact, some authorities recommend avoiding vitamin D supplements altogether. If you're not old, if your bones are strong, if you get adequate sunlight, and if you have a diet rich in vitamin D, many experts believe that you probably don't need a supplement.

As is the case with other vitamins, it's a good idea to check with your doctor before taking vitamin D supplements.

VITAMIN E

Vitamin E is a strong antioxidant. But do you need supplements or can you get enough in of it from food?

The case for supplements

The chorus in favor of vitamin E is a loud one:

- Says Carper, "There is virtually no way you can get enough vitamin E in food to protect cells against free radical damage and ward off heart disease, cancer, declining immunity, and other chronic diseases of aging."

- "Vitamin E is inexpensive and has no known side effects, and good authorities, such as the *Harvard Medical Letter*, support its use," writes Stanford University's James Fries in *Living Well.*

- Vitamin E supplements can apparently help the heart. The Harvard School of Public Health and Boston's Brigham and Women's Hospital conducted a study of more than 87,000 women and 40,000 men. The men who took vitamin E supplements had 35 to 40 percent fewer first-time cardiac problems than the non-vitamin takers; the women who took vitamin E had 40 to 50 percent less risk of heart disease than the women who didn't.

    Ford reports, "A 1993 study published in the New England Journal of Medicine reported that men and women taking a daily vitamin E supplement had 66 percent less risk of developing heart disease than a control group taking none."

    And Quebec's Laval University conducted a study in which men who ingested vitamin E supplements for a decade had 78 percent fewer deaths from heart disease than men who didn't.

- Vitamin E supplements can help to control cholesterol. Carper cites a study by Ishwarlal Jialal of the University of Texas Southwestern Medical Center, showing that vitamin E supplements "slashed LDL cholesterol oxidation—and thus its ability to foster artery damage and heart disease—[by] a dramatic 40 percent!"

- Vitamin E can fight atherosclerosis. Says Fries, "Recent data strongly suggest that vitamin E, 400 units per day, can reduce coronary atherosclerosis by 40 percent."

- Vitamin E can help to prevent stroke. In one study of women, vitamin E supplements reduced the risk of stroke by 54 percent, Ford reports.

- Vitamin E can raise immunity. Carper mentions a study by Simin Meydani, Ph.D., a nutritional immunologist at Tufts University. Doses of 400 or 800 IU per day, given to people over age 60, improved immunity "by 10 to 50 percent within thirty days."

- Vitamin E can fight cancer. The National Cancer Institute has discovered that taking 100 IU of vitamin E supplements (and other supplements) cut the risk of mouth and throat cancer in half. Carper cites a Yale University study in which vitamin E supplementation halved the risk of lung cancer in nonsmokers. She adds, "A recent study of 35,000 Iowa women found that those under age 65 who got the most vitamin E—largely from supplements—had a 68 percent lower chance of colon cancer."

The case against

A minority of authorities find vitamin E supplements—or at least some of the rosier claims made for them—to be worthless. Bortz, citing experiments on animals, says, "The hypothesis of a vitamin E fountain of youth hasn't held up."

Moreover, says Barnard, "My own recommendation is not to rely on supplements but rather to incorporate natural vitamin E-rich foods into an optimal menu."

But if, as most experts advocate, you choose to use vitamin E supplements . . .

Dosage

Most experts who recommend vitamin E recommend from 100 to 400 international units daily. Going far above that amount can hurt some people. The vitamin's power to slow blood coagulation (and thus hinder the development of strokes) can cause trouble if bleeding takes place. Barnard says, "People with bleeding disorders or high blood pressure may be advised by their doctors to avoid vitamin E." Carper warns, "In doses exceeding 400 IU, vitamin E . . . is not recommended in people taking anticoagulant drugs or facing surgery."

At doses of vitamin E well above 400 IU, fatal consequences can occur. Carper warns, "Toxicity can occur at over 3,200 IU daily."

But, Barnard says, "Such large doses are really used as medications rather than as part of normal nutrition, and they are not a guide to how much your body actually needs."

The bottom line for people who do take vitamin E (after consulting with their doctors, of course): keep the dosage within a safe range.

SPECIFIC SUPPLEMENTS: MINERALS

"A Chinese alchemist in the first century B.C. advised the Han emperor to transmute mercury into gold and make tableware from it," writes Hayflick. "By eating and drinking from these utensils, he would achieve immortality."

From that time on, a belief in the life-giving power of minerals would mark longevity research.

Hayflick continues, "Some of the Chinese alchemical thought was probably transmitted to the West by way of Arabic science." As *Search for Immortality* notes: "The Arabs . . . sought to find and isolate the universal agent, often called the philosopher's stone, with which all things—gold, youth, life itself—could be fashioned. One Arab name for this magical substance was *al iksir*, a term that survives in English as *elixir*."

By the thirteenth century, alchemy was the hot topic among Europe's longevity experimenters. Like the Chinese, they believed in a link between gold and long life. "Alchemists recommended consuming gold tinctures from gold cups," says Orlock.

While alchemy is gone, taking with it the belief in the life-extending power of gold, the belief in the benefits of other minerals remains. Many experts recommend taking supplements of calcium, selenium, zinc, and other elements.

Others disagree. "A diet featuring plant foods and some dairy products will easily satisfy all the known mineral requirements of the body," says Georgakas.

The next sections will cover the usefulness—or lack of it—in some of the most popular mineral supplements.

CALCIUM

Calcium can help strengthen bones and lower blood pressure; it may also fight colon cancer. Do you need supplements of calcium? "Yes—unless you religiously eat several servings a day of high calcium foods," Carper says. Such foods include milk, fish, nuts, beans, and dark-green leafy vegetables.

The likeliest candidates for calcium supplementation include anyone whose bones face large calcium losses, such as postmenopausal women or older people of either gender. In addition, anyone who doesn't eat several daily servings of high-calcium foods may benefit from supplements.

The experts recommend doses ranging from 500 to 2,000 milligrams per day, depending on your age, gender, and diet. For instance, older women who don't eat calcium-rich foods tend to need larger doses. The supplements should be taken with meals and spaced out over the day rather than all at once.

Some experts caution against taking supplements that are formulated from oyster shells, dolomite (a rocky mineral), or bone meal, because such souces can be high in lead. Instead, the experts recommend calcium citrate or calcium carbonate. Perhaps the best known form of calcium carbonate is the antacid Tums.

Beware overdoses of calcium. Doses of 2,500 milligrams or more may cause constipation or kidney stones. As *Live Longer, Live Better* says, "Although consuming an excessive amount of calcium is not a problem for most people, check with your doctor before taking a supplement."

CHROMIUM

Chromium, found in whole grains, broccoli, peanuts, mushrooms, and brewer's yeast, can help the body process sugar. Unfortunately, Ryback says, "of all the vitamins and minerals, chromium is more likely to be in short supply in the American diet than any other substance."

If you can't adjust your diet to include chromium-rich foods, the experts who recommend supplements advise taking 200 micrograms daily.

But more isn't necessarily better. Carper notes, "There's no reason for most people to go above 200 micrograms per day in a supplement." She cautions, "If you are diabetic, take chromium supplements only with a doctor's supervision because the mineral may alter insulin requirements."

IRON

"Probably the most commonly supplemented mineral is iron," Georgakas says.

There are good reasons for certain people to take iron supplements. Says Carper: "Menstruating women tend to lose iron regularly in blood flow and may need iron supplements. Also, children and adolescents often do not get enough iron."

For other people, though, iron supplements can promote the development of free radicals and atherosclerosis. Consequently, it's probably a good idea to avoid iron supplements altogether, unless your doctor prescribes them.

MAGNESIUM

Many Americans don't get enough magnesium. And that's a shame, because magnesium—found in nuts, grains, dark-green leafy vegetables, and other plant foods—is useful in preventing heart disease, helping the body process calcium, and fighting off osteoporosis.

The more magnesium in your diet, the less that you need from supplements. Depending on the amount of magnesium in your diet, recommended doses of magnesium supplements range from 200 to 1,000 milligrams per day.

Be cautious, though. Doses on the upper half of the scale can cause diarrhea; larger doses can even be toxic. People who have had kidney troubles or heart disease should probably avoid magnesium supplements altogether. And anyone contemplating taking magnesium should talk to a doctor first.

POTASSIUM

Potassium can help to control blood pressure. It's especially important for older people to get enough of this mineral, since the amount of potassium in the body declines with age.

But that doesn't mean that it should be supplemented. As Hayflick says, "I am unaware of any studies designed to show whether diets supplemented with potassium would reverse this trend [of potassium decline with age]."

Most experts recommend getting potassium from foods rather than from supplements. "Check with your doctor before taking potassium supplements," the *Age Erasers* books advise. "Too much may aggravate kidney problems." Mindell says, "Excess amounts (over 18 grams) can be toxic."

SELENIUM

Selenium fights cancer and heart disease. Selenium sounds good, and it is—but in supplements, it's controversial.

"I don't recommend [supplements] because selenium is very powerful," says Barnard. "A little too much, and it becomes poisonous." Moore, in *Life Span*, agrees: "Western diets contain more than adequate amounts of selenium, according to Barry Halliwell, a British biochemist and authority on free radicals."

But Barnard and Moore are in the minority. Ford speaks for several experts when he says, "In the quantities needed, [selenium is] best supplied by supplements."

Most experts who favor selenium recommend taking 50 to 200 micrograms per day. Higher doses can lower the body's immunity to disease, according to the *Age Erasers* books, and can cause liver damage, says Carper.

Since the amount of selenium in food is not uniform, check with your doctor about how much selenium you should take from supplements.

ZINC

Zinc, available in beans, poultry, eggs, oysters, and wheat germ, helps keep the immune system working. Unfortunately, Ford says, "The standard American diet remains deficient [in zinc]." It's likely to remain deficient, too. Carper explains, "It's difficult to get enough zinc in the diet, especially for vegetarians and people who are cutting back on meat."

If you don't get enough zinc in your diet, the authorities who recommend taking supplements suggest consuming 15 to 50 milligrams daily, with most recommending about 25 milligrams.

Use caution, though. Doses over 50 milligrams "can suppress immune functions and can have other detrimental effects," Carper warns.

Barnard issues the most solemn warning of all. "Zinc can be toxic," he says, "and should not be used unless specifically prescribed."

MULTIVITAMIN AND
MULTIMINERAL SUPPLEMENTS

Drug stores and natural-food stores often feature multivitamin—multi-mineral pills. Many experts advise taking them, and even those who condemn other supplements rarely come out strongly against them; the dose of any one element in the multis is usually too low to damage the body. As Orlock says, "Most researchers now agree that supplementing one's diet with a daily multivitamin probably won't hurt, and it just might help."

Among those people who should seriously consider taking multis are "anyone over 40 with a diet that does not meet the USDA's minimum food guide standards," says Ford. (As a reminder, he adds, "The guidelines are to eat at least six servings of whole grain cereals; two servings of fruit; three of vegetables; and at least one of legumes each day as well as a few nuts and seeds.")

What should you buy? *Staying Young* recommends a balanced vitamin and mineral supplement containing iron, zinc, copper, selenium, iodine, calcium, magnesium, vitamin A, the vitamin B group, vitamin C, vitamin D, and especially vitamin E and beta carotene. Carper notes that the Theragran-M brand seems effective.

One last note on multis. Bortz says: "A balanced multivitamin tablet or capsule should cost only a few cents. Also, I discourage the ultra high-potency formulas as unnecessary and almost always too expensive. Vitamins also lose shelf potency, so buy them fresh."

MEGADOSES

If supplements are controversial, megadoses of supplements are even more so. Megadoses are simply very large doses of various supplements. Many people take them, and some experts approve of them.

But more don't.

THE POSITIVE VIEW

"To best stave off aging, it's necessary to take megadoses of antioxidant vitamins and minerals," Carper says. UCLA research pathologist Steven Harris adds that even if taking supplements does no good, "the side effects are zip. It's kind of a gamble where the downside is absolutely nothing."

"I don't think that vitamin supplements or even megavitamin programs do much harm, as a rule," says Fries. "Generally, the potential harm of unneeded vitamin intake involves only the unnecessary cost of the vitamins and the possibility that needed medical care may not be undertaken because of the assumption that the vitamins are enough."

THE NEGATIVE VIEW

"Vitamins are like light switches," Bortz says. "You need a certain number to light your house. Following the same analogy, having 10 or 100 times that number doesn't make the lights any brighter. . . . There is no evidence that consumption of megavitamins improves exercise performance or has any beneficial effects on the aging process."

The *Age Erasers* books are blunter: "Forget super-supplements. You may see 'high potency' or 'extra strength' labels. These products typically contain levels of vitamins and minerals that . . . may be hazardous. . . . Or you may just be excreting the excess, in which case you're wasting your money."

What's more, observes *Live Longer, Live Better*, "Megadoses of any one vitamin may inhibit the absorption of other nutrients." DiGiovanna adds that megadosing "can lead to additional malnutrition, toxicity, and serious or life-threatening malfunction or failure of many body systems."

Why do these problems happen? DiGiovanna explains: "Because of age-related decreases in mechanisms, such as nutrient storage, conversion, and excretion, that permit adaptation to excess materials; and [because of] the likelihood that excess nutrients will aggravate the existing problems or cause new ones in weakened organs or systems."

So if the body isn't in strong youthful shape, megadosing can kill it.

Another reason for the anti-megadose wave is uncertainty. Walford, who recommends supplements, believes that all of the research on taking huge doses is not in yet: "This lack of pertinent scientific data does not justify indiscriminate megadosing of vitamins, minerals, or other supplements."

Consequently, writes Michael Fossel in *Reversing Human Aging*, large doses may deliver as-yet-unsuspected diseases, especially over long periods: "Given enough time . . . the side effects of high doses might become noticeable and even fatal. . . . Perhaps the slight detrimental effects of vitamin C on kidney function—stone formation, for example—[may] become overwhelming after taking large doses regularly for 50 years."

The advice to check with your doctor before taking supplements goes double for megadoses.

GLANDS AND HORMONES

ACCORDING TO HAYFLICK, HORMONE THERAPY IS MORE THAN A century old. "In 1889, when he was 72, the eminent French physiologist Charles-Edouard Brown-Sequard reported that he had rejuvenated his health by inoculating extracts of crushed domestic animal testicles into his arms and legs. Over the next several years, he and thousands of other physicians inoculated many older people. . . . The cult of injection spread throughout the world."

Too bad that Brown-Sequard was wrong. "No one regained his lost youth and potency from Sequardienne treatments," says *Search for Immortality*.

Still, Hayflick finds a happy ending: "Although the extract prepared by Brown-Sequard has been proven to be ineffective, he is given credit for drawing attention to the use of tissue and glandular extracts as the sources of important therapeutic agents. He is considered to be the father of endocrinology [the study of glands and hormones]."

Others would follow in Brown-Sequard's optimistic—if misguided—tracks:

- In the late 1890s, some men tried injections or grafts from monkey and goat testicles. "What might have been another amusing, if expensive, example of human gullibility became tragic when one set of grafts inadvertently used syphilitic monkeys, transferring that disease to humans at a time when penicillin had not yet been discovered," says Georgakas.

- In the 1920s, Hayflick says, "John R. 'Doc' Brinkley became a millionaire by transplanting the glands from goats and other animals into thousands of old people. . . . Goats were chosen as testicle donors because of Brinkley's belief that they were sexual athletes."

  Search for Immortality continues the story: "On a good day, 500 people would swarm in . . . seeking rejuvenation at the doctor's hands. . . . In 1930, however, the business that had reportedly made him a millionaire began to unravel. . . . In 1941, the doctor retired from practice . . . and declared bankruptcy."

- In 1918, *Search for Immortality* reports, physician Serge Voronoff (sometimes spelled Veronoff) "began transplanting bits of chimpanzee and monkey testes onto the genitals of elderly men. More than 1,000 patients underwent the costly 'monkey gland treatment.'"

  Following in a familiar pattern, notes Hayflick, "Voronoff's early claims were soon disproven, and his method was abandoned."

- "In the 1920s and 1930s, prison doctors at California's San Quentin penitentiary implanted the testicles of executed felons into thirty prisoners in an effort to increase virility and stem the aging process," says Hayflick. "In view of the laws of immunology, which were discovered later, these transplants must have been uniformly rejected by the recipients."

Although these attempts failed, hormone supplements may be useful in other ways and may yet be important in extending life. After all, hormone levels do fall as people age, so replacing them may help to replace lost youth.

They remain controversial, though. The advocates of hormone supplements say that hormones can raise immunity levels and help people to live longer. But in April 1997, the federal government's National Institute on Aging warned that hormones can have some ugly side effects, including high blood pressure, diabetes, and cancer.

Before you head to a health food store or pharmacy to get hormone tablets, check with your doctor. In the meantime, here are some notes on specific hormones.

ESTROGEN

"[Women] on estrogen replacement therapy live three years longer, on average, than those who are not," says *Aging on Hold*.

"On average" is a tricky term. Women on ERT also run severe medical risks.

BENEFITS

What can estrogen do?

- In a 16-year study at Brigham and Women's Hospital, concluded in 1997, women on estrogen supplements had a 37 percent lower risk of death than women not taking estrogen. The risk of death by heart disease in particular was cut approximately in half.

- Estrogen replacement can battle osteoporosis and slow the loss of bone, resulting in bones that are less easily broken. The American Geriatrics Society explains, "There is a 50 percent reduction in the risk of hip and wrist fractures in women who use estrogen."

- Estrogen can help the brain. A study of 1,000 women aged 70 and up, conducted at the Columbia University School of Public Health, found that women on estrogen replacement reduced their risk of Alzheimer's disease by up to 40 percent.

RISKS

Still, says Bortz, "taking estrogen is a mixed blessing." Depression, gall bladder problems, headaches, and weight gain are among its possible drawbacks.

But the most deadly risk of estrogen replacement is cancer.

- "Women age 60 to 66 on hormone replacement therapy have an 87 percent increased risk of breast cancer," Mindell says.

- Dr. Brian Walsh of the Menopause Clinic at Brigham and Women's Hospital believes, "Taking estrogen alone increases a woman's risk for endometrial [uterus-lining] cancer about fourfold." A Brigham and Women's Hospital study on estrogen found that women who took supplements for a decade or longer had a risk of dying from breast cancer that was 43 percent higher than that of women not taking estrogen.

YES OR NO?

Mindell asks, "Should breast cancer be the price we pay for reduced risk of heart disease and bone fractures?" He answers, "No." And Barnard says that estrogen causes more problems than it solves.

But a slight majority of longevity authorities who address the issue favor estrogen replacement. Dr. Fran Kaiser of St. Louis University Medical School points out, "One out of two women after menopause has the risk of a heart attack, while one out of nine to twelve has the risk of breast cancer." You may not mind increasing an 11 percent risk of breast cancer in order to shrink the 50 percent risk of heart disease.

To make an informed decision, *Age Erasers for Women* advocates finding a good doctor, knowing your family history (if your family is free of breast cancer but has a long record of heart disease, then estrogen therapy may pose few risks and many benefits), and asking others about their use of the therapy ("talk to other women your age . . . about their thinking, decisions, and experiences surrounding [hormone replacement]").

If you choose estrogen replacement, keep an eye out for cancer. To catch possible cancer early, perform a monthly breast self-examination, get a mammogram, and obtain an endometrial biopsy, which examines the lining of the uterus for cancer.

To reduce estrogen's risks, DiGiovanna recommends "using small doses of estrogen, administering estrogen by injection rather than orally, [and] administering estrogen in cycles that mimic natural cycles."

ESTROGEN PLUS PROGESTERONE

Adding the ovarian hormone progesterone to estrogen is another way to lower the risk of cancer—specifically uterine cancer.

Proponents of progesterone injections range from true believers ("Combining [estrogen] with progesterone," says Orlock, "overcomes this risk [of uterine cancer]") to the qualifiers and hedgers ("The long-term benefits are unclear, but studies to date indicate that the combination is safer than estrogen alone . . . if a woman still has her uterus," *Live Longer, Live Better* reports). Despite these differences, a rough pro-progesterone consensus does seem to exist.

Still, progesterone has problems. Bortz says, "Progesterone offsets some of the protective effect of the estrogen"—that is, it lowers estrogen's protection against heart disease and other maladies. Don't expect it to be a panacea.

ESTROGEN PLUS PROGESTIN

Another well-known technique is adding the synthetic hormone progestin to estrogen. Together, progestin and estrogen may actually outdo estrogen at its own game. *Age Erasers for Women* says, "A large study of 15,800 people from four areas of the country . . . estimated that women who took estrogen alone decreased their risk of heart disease . . . and that women who used estrogen with progestin would have even greater benefit."

But progestin generates its own controversies. According to *Age Erasers for Women*, "There's some question among researchers about whether progestin reduces the protective effect of estrogen."

In fact, writes health journalist Jessica Snyder Sachs in *Weight Watchers* magazine, progestin might actually raise the risk of cancer. "The most definitive research to date, the Nurses' Health Study at Harvard Medical School in Boston, found a 40 percent increased risk [of cancer] in women taking the estrogen–progestin combination and a slightly lower risk in women on estrogen alone."

Age Erasers for Women advises, "You and your doctor need to weigh the pros and cons before deciding whether estrogen alone or in combination with progestin"—or, for that matter, with progesterone— "is right for you."

WOMEN AT RISK

For some women, deciding whether or not to use estrogen is easy. Women who have liver disease, clotting disorders such as phlebitis, risk factors for breast cancer (especially a personal or family history of the disease), or blood-vessel problems (such as varicose veins or high blood pressure) should avoid estrogen supplements entirely.

DHEA

The hormone dehydroepiandrosterone—alias DHEA—has been touted as a miracle formula:

- In *Biological Anthropology*, Solomon Katz, Ph.D., of the University of Pennsylvania and David Armstrong, Ph.D., of Gallaudet University point out that the gene for DHEA "is substantially implicated in the development of the biological substrates of longevity."

- Chopra, in *Ageless Body, Timeless Mind*, notes, "Higher DHEA is also associated with longer survival and decreased death from all diseases in older men."

- In his book *Development, Aging, and Disease*, Vladimir Dilman of New York University Medical Center says plainly, "DHEA is a key anti-aging substance."

WHAT IS DHEA?

DHEA is a hormone that the adrenal gland produces in large quantities. In fact, it's one of the most common hormones in the body. "It appears to block the destructive effects of stress on the immune system," Orlock says.

But as a body ages, its DHEA levels fall, often with fatal results. "Low DHEA levels have been linked to heart attacks and increased vulnerability to some cancers," says Orlock.

What makes DHEA especially interesting to longevity scientists is this: "Its levels decline with age in a fairly linear fashion," says Ford. In fact, says Chopra, "it is the only hormone that declines in a straight line with age." Moreover, says Fossel, "Its congenital absence is apparently fatal."

So losing DHEA may cause aging. Therefore, replacing it may reverse the course of aging and extend life. At least that's what one scientist hoped.

DHEA EXPERIMENTS

In his book *The Clock of Ages*, the University of Washington's John Medina writes, "Etienne-Emile Baulieu, M.D., at the Krelmin-Bicetre hospital in Paris . . . [discovered that] when small doses [of DHEA] were administered daily, there was increased mobility, less joint pain, more restful sleep, a greater sense of psychological well-being"—attributes common in long-lived people— "and many other characteristics of aging reversal."

What's more, studies of DHEA replacement have found beneficial effects involving cholesterol levels, body fat and obesity, cancer (particularly breast cancer), heart and artery disease, bone strength, immunity, and other bodily functions ranging from mental abilities to muscle power.

THE GREAT UNKNOWNS

Before you start taking DHEA, be aware that it carries a lot of mysteries:

- According to journalist Gail Sheehy, DHEA researcher Samuel Yen, a University of California endocrinologist, "[was] the first to point out that no one knows what is the proper dose . . . or how men and women differ in utilizing it."

- DHEA use may cause side effects, from beard growth and endometrial cancer in women to liver damage and possibly even prostate cancer in men.

- DHEA replacement may not actually cause the great effects for which it has been praised. Hayflick notes that mice who were fed DHEA lived longer than those that weren't. But the DHEA mice, he says, tended to eat less than usual. "Some biogerontologists believed that the increase in longevity attributed to DHEA may instead be a manifestation of the longevity-extending effect of caloric restriction."

DHEA experiments continue. If you want to try it, it is available, but ask your doctor to examine the most current research on the subject.

MELATONIN

As you age, your body produces less of the hormone melatonin, which regulates the body's cycle of sleeping and waking. Melatonin is sold as a natural sleep aid.

How does melatonin enter into longevity? The process starts, naturally enough, at melatonin's source, the pineal gland.

Italian doctor Walter Pierpaoli transplanted the pineal glands of young mice into old ones. The old mice not only lived to the far end of their maximum life span; they also did it in robust health.

Transplants may not be necessary. Pierpaoli also put melatonin in the drinking water of lab mice. The mice lived about six months longer than normal—a span that's equivalent to at least fifteen years in humans.

HOW IT MAY EXTEND LIFE

Melatonin has been given credit for everything but putting out the cat at night. As journalist Jessica Snyder Sachs writes, "Claims for melatonin run the gamut from cancer prevention to improved immune system functioning and increased vitality and longevity."

SIDE EFFECTS

Here some trouble begins. Melatonin can affect the mind and the emotions. Among its reported side effects are depression and nightmares.

And although it has extended life in aging rats, "melatonin reduces longevity in young rats, so people might be unwise to use it regularly before hitting age 40," writes journalist Peter Doskoch in *Psychology Today*. "The effects of long-term use are unknown."

Harvard Medical School's Steven Reppert and David Weaver wrote in a 1995 issue of the scientific journal *Cell* that some melatonin treatments on experimental animals "actually shortened survival by inducing reproductive tract tumors."

And, writes Sheehy, consuming too much melatonin can "cripple the natural production of the glands of [the overdosers'] own bodies."

NOW WHAT?

Despite Pierpaoli's encouraging experiments on rodents, there's little confirmed evidence that melatonin can extend the life of humans. But if it does turn out to help raise immunity or fight cancer, supplements of melatonin may be useful someday. If you want to dose yourself, check with your doctor first.

OTHER SUBSTANCES

SOD AND CATALASE

The enzymes superoxide dismutase (SOD) and catalase have been touted as life stretchers. Research into these substances offers intriguing possibilities for extending life and health. Bottles of SOD and catalase tablets line the shelves of health-food stores.

THE GOOD NEWS—AND THE CATCH

Live Longer, Live Better says that SOD may be "a key to longevity." Fossel is more scientific but no less sanguine, defining SOD as "a common antioxidant protein that is important to the aging process."

SOD is an enzyme that cells produce to turn free radicals into less harmful substances, thus diminishing the power of free radicals to damage the body. Evidence of the power of SOD to extend life comes from Banaras Hindu University's M.S. Kanungo, who writes in his book *Genes and Aging*, "Longer-lived species have higher levels of SOD." The University of Wales's Denis Bellamy notes in *Ageing: A Biomedical Perspective*, that humans have more SOD than apes, which have more than monkeys, which have more than rodents—and humans live longer than apes, which outlive monkeys, which outlive rodents.

Like SOD, catalase is one of "[the] major enzymes fueling the [body's] antioxidant machinery," according to Carper. The two enzymes, working with a third enzyme, glutathione peroxidase, "not only trap but metabolize free radicals," Fossel explains. "Starting with an unpaired oxygen atom, for example, these enzymes can produce innocuous and useful molecules, such as water."

It sounds as if popping SOD and catalase pills should help the body eliminate free radicals and live longer. Unfortunately, that's not true. When you consume catalase or SOD, the stomach's gastric juices break it down into its component molecules and destroy it. Even if you take several SOD or catalase pills, your body won't be able to use them.

There may be edible forms of these substances available in the future—but don't bother with the ones on the market today.

GLUTATHIONE

"One of the most important antioxidants produced in the body," is how Mindell describes glutathione. *Aging on Hold* dubs it "[part of] the cell's arsenal against free radicals."

What is glutathione?

- Barnard calls it "the carrier molecule that hauls toxins out of the body."

- Mindell says, "Glutathione may help protect against cancer, radiation poisoning, and the detrimental effects of cigarette smoke and alcohol abuse."

- "Glutathione fortifies cells in the GI [gastrointestinal] tract, providing a barrier against the free-radical-producing fats," Carper explains.

What if you don't have much glutathione? "Low levels of serum glutathione have been associated with cell damage, depressed immunity, and premature aging," Mindell says.

"Glutathione is a popular supplement in Japan, the country with the longest life span in the world," says Mindell. Supplements of glutathione may contribute to the health of the immune system as it gets older, according to the Human Nutrition Research Center on Aging at Tufts University.

While glutathione is available in fruits and vegetables, the experts who recommend supplements of any substance say that you should take 40 to 100 milligrams of glutathione daily. Taking more isn't widely recommended at this time.

COENZYME Q-10

Enzymes such as SOD and catalase can cause chemical changes within cells. Coenzymes work with them. Coenzyme Q-10, says Mindell, "is found in every cell in the body and is essential in facilitating the process that provides cells with energy." Heart surgeon Robert Willix, in his book *Healthy at 100*, calls coenzyme Q-10 "a naturally occurring antioxidant."

What does this coenzyme do?

- "It preserves youth in laboratory animals," says Carper. "It is thought to have particular energy-stimulating effects on heart muscle cells and has long been used in Europe and Japan to treat heart failure."

- Mindell calls Q-10 "very effective in preventing toxicity from a large number of drugs used to treat cancer, high blood pressure, and other diseases."

Those who recommend supplements advise taking 20 to 30 milligrams of Q-10 per day.

Can more be dangerous? "Even at very high doses, no significant toxicity in animal or long-term human studies has been recorded," Carper says. Dr. L. Stephen Coles of the California Institute of Technology agrees, "There is no downside to taking CoQ-10."

Nevertheless, it's probably safest to check with your doctor before taking coenzyme Q-10.

OMEGA-3 FATTY ACIDS

Omega-3 fatty acids, found in fish, are among the few fats that longevity experts actually like. Omega-3s help to keep the arteries open, fight cholesterol, and lower triglyceride levels.

Since omega-3s are found in fish, many people take fish oil supplements, sold at health-food stores. Carper cites the advice of Alexander Leaf, M.D., of Harvard University's School of Public Health: "It's OK to take up to a gram (1,000 milligrams) of omega-3 fish oil daily in capsules." Carper and Walford recommend the dietary supplement MaxEpa as a good source of fish oil.

But *Live Longer, Live Better* warns, "Fish oil supplements are not a good source of omega-3; in some cases, they may even be harmful." Omega-3s inhibit blood clotting, so they're not recommended for people who have problems involving clotting or bleeding.

Whether or not you have clotting problems, every expert—even those who recommend taking omega-3 or fish-oil supplements—advises checking with your doctor before taking a supplement.

DRUGS

"A HUGE NUMBER OF PREVENTABLE AGING PROBLEMS CAN BE TRACED to the indiscriminate use of prescription drugs," Chopra says. For example:

- "[A] study recently published in *The Journal of the American Medical Association* found that close to 25 percent of all Americans over 65 were given prescriptions for medications that were either unsafe or ineffective for the elderly," Mindell reports. "Many of the drugs that are routinely prescribed for older people are not designed for an aging body and often interact badly with other medications."

• Fries notes in *Living Well*: "In the senior years, prescription drugs are a more frequent cause of [life-shortening] impairment than alcohol or street drugs. Codeine, Valium, and a whole range of sedatives and tranquilizers can alter reflexes and judgment enough to cause accidents."

CHECKING THE MEDS

Before accepting medication, find out everything that you can about its effects. In particular, always ask your doctor:

• What are the medication's side effects?

• Can the medication interact with any other medication that I am taking?

• Do I take the medication with food or on an empty stomach?

Here are some notes involving these questions:

SIDE EFFECTS

The American Geriatrics Society notes, "Aging tends to increase our vulnerability to side effects." In fact, says Fries, "Somewhere between 10 and 20 percent of hospital admissions for seniors are the direct result of medication side effects."

MIXING AND MATCHING

"As a pharmacist," Mindell says, "I believe that no more than three drugs should be taken simultaneously to avoid interactions or side effects, and that includes over-the-counter medications."

The American Geriatrics Society explains, "One drug may either cause another to act more powerfully or may inhibit its action." Such problems increase as the number of drugs ingested or the age of the person taking them rises.

"If you must take several drugs simultaneously, be sure that you are being closely monitored by your physician," Mindell advises.

ASPIRIN

Of all the drugs taken to extend life or simply to make you feel better, the most commonly used is probably aspirin. Among the claims made for this familiar little pill:

- Aspirin fights heart disease. "A Harvard Nurses' Health Study that tracked more than 121,000 nurses for fifteen years found that women who took one to six aspirin tablets per week cut their risk of heart attack by 30 percent," *Age Erasers for Women* reports. In both men and women, aspirin can lessen the rate of death from heart disease in people who have already had a heart attack.

- Aspirin fights cancer. The American Cancer Society examined more than 600,000 people. The ones who ingested aspirin at least sixteen times monthly were half as likely to get colon cancer as those who didn't take aspirin. Aspirin "may also have a similar benefit on other digestive tract cancers such as those of the esophagus, stomach, and rectum, says *Live Longer, Live Better.*

WHO NEEDS ASPIRIN?

Anyone with diabetes, high blood pressure, or high cholesterol levels. Also, people who have suffered heart attacks or who have a family history of heart disease. Men, particularly men over 50, are prime candidates for the little pill.

DOSAGE

"Just how much aspirin you should take," the *Age Erasers* books say, "remains debatable."

Daily recommendations range from *Live Longer, Live Better*'s 30 milligrams ("a little less than half a baby aspirin") to the *Age Erasers* books' three regular aspirin (about 900 to 975 milligrams). Your doctor can prescribe the right dose (if any) for you.

But don't overdose. Extra aspirin doesn't seem to bring better results. What's more, says Georgakas, "in doses of 20 to 30 grams, it is lethal."

DANGERS

According to many experts, you should avoid aspirin if you have a bleeding disorder, an ulcer, high blood pressure, or a problem of the kidney or liver. One reason for this caution: "Regular use of aspirin will lead to internal bleeding," Georgakas says. Such bleeding is especially serious in two areas—the stomach and the brain.

"Aspirin can be very irritating to the stomach and can cause bleeding and ulcers in some people," Mindell says. The symptoms can get worse over the years. "As [you] age," writes Fries in *Living Well*, "aspirin becomes more irritating to your stomach." "People on aspirin should be closely monitored by their physicians for gastrointestinal bleeding or other problems," Mindell recommends.

And for the brain, aspirin is both good and bad.

THE STROKE CONTROVERSY

If you have already had a stroke, aspirin may help to prevent another one. "Aspirin," says the American Geriatrics Society, can "help prevent TIAs [transient ischemic attacks, small strokes that last less than a day] and subsequent strokes. Aspirin reduces the risk of stroke due to carotid artery disease from approximately 19 to 12 percent over a three-year period."

But, says *Staying Young*, "There may be little or no benefit to taking aspirin to prevent a first stroke." The *Age Erasers* books agree: "Unless you already have a risk factor, such as atherosclerosis or a prior stroke, it may not do you much good."

Aspirin can actually bring on strokes. This finding may seem to contradict the claim that aspirin can prevent strokes, but there are different kinds of strokes. While some strokes, such as TIAs, are caused by blood clots in the head—and aspirin can help to eliminate such clots—other strokes, known as hemorrhagic strokes, are caused by bleeding in the brain. And aspirin itself may increase the chance of such bleeding.

WHAT TO DO?

Let the experts explain:

"Do not take aspirin on a regular basis without first checking with your physician," Mindell advises.

"No one should consider taking aspirin regularly without consulting a physician," *Live Longer* recommends.

"You should not take aspirin to protect your heart without first consulting your doctor," advises *Staying Young*.

"Be sure to obtain your doctor's approval before taking aspirin on a daily basis," Walford says.

"See your doctor before you start an aspirin regimen for stroke prevention," advise the *Age Erasers* books.

DOING WITHOUT

One strategy that the longevity literature mentions occasionally is doing without drugs altogether—or at least using them as little as possible. Chopra notes that in psychiatrist Stephen Jewett's 1973 survey of people in their late eighties and above, the subjects "used less medication in their lifetimes than many [other] people use in a week."

Given the problems that drugs can cause, Jewett's oldsters may be onto something. "Use as few drugs as possible," Fries recommends. "When any new problem arises [in the body], suspect first that it might be the result of a drug you are taking. This is the easiest of all medical problems to treat. You stop the drug, and generally the problem goes away."

Instead of drugs, Fries advises, "use life-style change." For instance, "avoiding salt in your diet is better than taking a [so-called] water pill. Exercise programs can reduce the need for blood pressure medications, and weight reduction will usually work better than pills for diabetes."

In fact, "You should always ask yourself whether elimination of all medicine might be possible," Fries says. "If you think this might be feasible, then talk it over with your doctor. At the least, you and your doctor may develop a plan that involves fewer medications, even if they cannot all be eliminated."

Fries's advice seems sensible. It is so easy for drugs to be misused—by accidental overdose, in dangerous combination with other drugs, and by other means—that if you and your doctor favor pulling back from a drug or two, it may be worth a try.

THE FUTURE
PART SIX:

WHY DO WE AGE AND DIE? AND HOW CAN WE STOP OR DELAY THAT PROCESS?

There is no universally accepted answer. Several theories that are duking it out for primacy offer the basis for what may be a triumph for longevity. If science can identify and understand the process that causes aging and death—or at least the most important of several processes—then the world may be able to take a big step closer to erasing that process and thereby extending life.

THEORIES OF ACCUMULATION

ERROR ACCUMULATION/ ERROR CATASTROPHE THEORY

As you age, your body makes mistakes—and keeps making them. That's one of the ideas behind error theory. In *The Clock of Ages*, the University of Washington's John Medina writes: "This theory rests on the assumption that as cells get older, they accumulate errors. These errors collect possibly due to the normal wear and tear of living within a sometimes hostile planet (scientists call these *environmental insults*)."

In his book *Human Aging*, DiGiovanna explains: "Damage to the genes has little effect at first. However, after many years . . . damaged molecules spread increasing numbers of mistakes throughout the cell and the body." Hayflick writes in *How and Why We Age*, "[The] faults in various molecules accumulate to a point where metabolic failures occur, resulting in age changes and, finally, death."

HOW WELL DOES THIS THEORY SCORE?

Says Hayflick: "Error theories have much to recommend them, and the expectation is that they will continue to be modified as new data accumulate. In the future, there is a good chance that some version of an error theory will turn out to explain an important proportion of age changes."

ACCUMULATION OF MUTATIONS/
SOMATIC MUTATION

Similar to the error theory, the theory of somatic mutations was so named because it affects the body's somatic cells. The somatic cells are the ones that reproduce and die. (Other cells, the germ cells, don't work this way; they effectively live until the body dies.)

"The somatic mutation theory proposes that harmful factors from the environment (e.g., radiation, toxic chemicals) injure the genes," DiGiovanna explains. So far, this theory resembles the error theories.

But while the error theories focus on cell damage as a problem in itself, mutation theories maintain that such damage causes genetic mutations, which are "passed on to the next generation of cells when the cell divides" (according to Ricklefs and Finch in *Aging: A Natural History*).

The problem, says Kanungo, author of *Genes and Aging*, is that these mutations can destroy genes and chromosomes. Mutations can also change genes, with ugly effects. "Mutated genes can create havoc with the body's proteins," say Ricklefs and Finch in *Aging: A Natural History*.

Since proteins are crucial to just about every function—they form the foundation of muscles and tissues, and regulate genes and chemical reactions within the body—mutations can mean trouble. According to Kanungo: "Cell death occurs when the mutation load in a cell increases beyond a critical level. So the number of . . . cells decreases, and the overall functional ability of the organism declines."

And if an organism can't function, it dies.

HOLES IN THE THEORY

Says Kanungo, "Even though DNA damage may contribute to the aging process in certain tissues, neither the damage nor the failure to repair the damage is a direct cause of aging." *Aging: A Natural History* notes, "There is no doubt that changes in DNA do occur during aging, but the consequences are not clear."

"Evidence for the mutation and error theories is weak," adds Hayflick, "and their popularity, though quite high a decade or two ago, has declined significantly in recent years."

In other words, error accumulation and somatic mutation are great theories, but there aren't enough facts to back them up—at least not yet.

GLYCATION AND COLLAGEN CROSS-LINKING

This theory is all about sugar. When sugar enters the body, it binds to proteins. According to UCLA's Walford, writing in *The Anti-Aging Plan*, the sugar ends up "permanently altering [the proteins'] molecular structure. The proteins gradually turn yellow-brown, and their function is impaired. This process is called glycation." *Aging: A Natural History* notes that hemoglobin (red blood) as well as collagen and elastin, "molecules that compose the connective tissues in our joints and elsewhere," can become glycated.

If too much tissue becomes glycated and suffers from impaired function, it can hurt, age, or kill the entire organism—so the theory says.

"The ultimate products of [glycation] have been called Advanced Glycosylation End-products (AGE)," says Hayflick. Like sugars, AGEs can attach themselves to proteins—but they can cause other damage as well.

AGEs can cause nearby molecules to cross-link with each other. "[Cross-linking] refers to the hardening of connective tissues, and has been likened to cells that are glued together or toughened in the way [that] leather is in tanning," *Aging: A Natural History* explains.

DiGiovanna says, "Cross-linkage theories maintain that [cross-linking] inhibits the movement of materials and parts of the body, resulting in malfunctioning and aging."

One of the proteins hit hardest by cross-linking is collagen, "the body's most abundant fiber" (as Carol Orlock calls it in *The End of Aging*). "[Cross-linked] collagen . . . may impede metabolic processes by obstructing the passage of nutrients and wastes into and out of cells," Orlock notes.

And so, Georgakas reports in *The Methuselah Factors*, "The hardened connective tissue becomes less able to deliver oxygen, nutrients, hormones, and other substances to the cells." The result: impaired function and, possibly, aging and death.

Unfortunately, Georgakas says, "No enzyme or other substance has yet been found to combat cross-linkage." But, Walford says, "We can to some extent reduce the progress of glycation."

How? "By avoiding the eating habits that produce high glucose values." The most direct way is to avoid sugars.

BUT IS IT TRUE?

Hayflick debunks cross-linking: "There is little doubt that cross-linking occurs in collagen and some other proteins, but the idea that it occurs in the DNA of live, aging animals is only speculation. . . . Even if it does occur, there is no good experimental evidence that it actually impedes metabolic processes or causes the formation of faulty molecules."

Hayflick concludes: "Perhaps cross-linking is only one of the many biochemical changes that occur over time and that contribute to the various aspects of aging—[but] it does not seem to be the most important contributor."

Still, no one has actually disproved the glycation and collagen cross-linking theories. More research will need to be conducted before anyone can definitively assess their importance.

WASTE PRODUCT THEORIES

Waste product theories, also known as clinker theories, involve the accumulation of waste products inside the body while the cells go about the business of being alive. Georgakas explains, "Cellular interactions produce unneeded by-products sometimes referred to as intercellular sludge, cellular garbage, [or] clinkers."

How does waste kill? "Viewed as a group, clinkers may be seen as so much corrosion or dust interfering with the delicate settings of the internal biological clocks," Georgakas says. "If cells accumulate more waste than they can dispose of efficiently, a kind of cellular constipation results," Hayflick adds. "In time, so the theory goes, the accumulated toxins and refuse could hamper normal cell function and slowly kill the cell."

If enough cells are killed, the entire organism will die.

ELIMINATING THE WASTE

There's no foolproof, universally accepted way to get rid of clinkers. "Various vitamins and antioxidants in combination with low-fat diets are being investigated to determine which would be most effective in preventing the accumulation of the garbage in the first place, in escorting the debris out of the body or in chemically transforming it into more useful compounds," Georgakas explains.

ELIMINATING-THE-WASTE THEORY

Some students of longevity doubt this hypothesis. "It is not clear whether these [waste products] should be thought of as causes or products of aging," says Georgakas.

"As attractive as the waste-product theory might be, there simply is no good evidence that the presence of [some wastes] actually interferes with normal cell function," Hayflick says. "Despite its indisputable presence in some old cells, few biogerontologists believe that [waste] plays a key role in the aging process."

As with other theories, the final word has yet to be written on this one.

WEAR AND TEAR

According to this theory, the thousand natural shocks that the flesh incurs are responsible for aging and death. "Theories of wear and tear," Georgakas explains, "hold that the body is aged, for the most part, by relentless outside pressures. These hostile forces include emotional factors, physical collisions, and environmental pollutants of every description."

Wear and tear obviously takes place. Muscles atrophy, joints get damaged, and body functions decline. Says Orlock: "When enough parts [of the body] have broken and can no longer be repaired—with medication, for example, or [by] transplants—the machine must be discarded. It dies."

FLAWS IN THE THEORY

Orlock points out that the human body doesn't always follow the normal rules of wear and tear. According to wear and tear theory, every time you use the human body—that is, every time you exercise—it should suffer wear and tear. In actuality, it becomes more resistant. It actually lasts longer the more you use it.

Besides, if wear and tear actually did cause a decline in function, people living for twenty to twenty-five years should have accumulated that many years of wear and tear and be in worse shape than when they were born. But they're not; most people in their early twenties are at the peak of health.

Finally, Hayflick says that even if wear and tear is an outward sign of aging, "[it might] have nothing to do with the fundamental causes of aging."

The theory is tempting, but it's not yet proven.

THEORIES OF PROGRAMMED DEATH

THE BODY MAY HAVE A SCHEDULE FOR ENDING ITS LIFE. THE IDEA MAY sound absurd, but it's the foundation for some respected theories.

THE HAYFLICK LIMIT

Leonard Hayflick—the same Hayflick quoted in these pages—is famous in longevity circles for a startling discovery: cells will divide only a limited number of times. The maximum number of times that a cell can divide is called the Hayflick limit.

The higher the Hayflick limit, the longer an organism lives. Short-lived creatures such as mice and rats have short Hayflick limits, while humans have long ones. Human cells can divide about fifty times before quitting.

Orlock says, "Once the reproducing cell approaches its limit, it takes longer to divide." The amount of time between doublings grows longer and longer, until finally the cell stops doubling altogether. At that point, Orlock continues, "The cell . . . begins to shrink. It fragments and decays. Then the cell dies."

When enough cells die, the organism in which they live begins to suffer. "Many older people have almost run out of [living] cells; there may be insufficient cells to function well," Fossel explains in *Reversing Human Aging*. "No longer can they fend off infection and trauma."

And if a body can't fend off infection and trauma, it dies.

THE IMPLICATIONS

If the Hayflick limit determines how long an organism can live, then extending the Hayflick limit may extend life.

At least, that's the theory. Georgakas explains: "Hayflick's work opens the possibility of . . . cellular transplants to fight disease and extend life. Cells that have completed only some of their potential divisions could be taken from an individual and kept in cold storage. At a later date, the cells could be returned to the donor to complete their pairings. Although there would be a finite limit to this process, life spans could be extended considerably longer than is now possible."

A HOLE IN THE THEORY

Orlock says, "While the typical cell may divide only 50 or 60 times, that's plenty of divisions to support a life span beyond the century range. If we lived as long as our cells allowed, we could all enjoy our maximum 120 years, and perhaps more."

Since the body actually dies before its cells reach full numbers of divisions, there may be more at work in aging and dying than the Hayflick limit. The limit clearly exists, but it may be only one of the possible causes of a body's death.

GENETIC PROGRAM ACTIVATION/
GENETIC CLOCK THEORY

Puberty usually arrives on schedule. So do menopause, the graying of hair, and the loss of baby teeth. Whether you're healthy or sick, your body determines when all these things happen.

And it may determine when aging and death happen, too.

At least one life process definitely involves death: a fetus's development of fingers and toes. Hayflick explains: "The tissue composing those regions starts as a single mass of cells, but the cells in the areas that become the spaces between the digits are destined to die. In this way, discrete fingers and toes are formed."

Since a genetic clock actually does tell fetal cells to die, then a genetic clock may tell the aging body to die. If so, perhaps there's a way to reset the clock, keep the cells going and live longer.

LOOPHOLES

The existence of suicidal genes contradicts the theory of evolution. Since our ancient ancestors died fairly young, "there were never enough old members of a species around, and none for a long enough time, to allow evolution to directly select for aging processes," says Hayflick.

And, according to DiGiovanna, "No one has been able to identify these [suicidal] genes."

So the theory remains just that—a theory.

OTHER
THEORIES

GENETIC ENGINEERING

Genetic engineering isn't exactly a theory. Scientists have already modified the genes of lower forms of life. In fact, researchers at Southern Methodist University have modified fruit fly genes in ways that increase the ability of the flies to fight off free radicals—and the modified flies lived longer than ordinary fruit flies.

As for humans, says *Search for Immortality*, "Some scientists believe the future of life extension lies in manipulating the genetic blueprint."

"The primary site of aging is the genome," says Kanungo in *Genes and Aging*. The genome is the entire bank of genes for a species. And it's being mapped.

"The Genome Project, which is intended to identify the exact location of every human gene, is scheduled to be completed by the year 2005," Orlock explains. "Even as it progresses, other researchers are trying to identify protective genes by backtracking from the damage that genes cause—in heart disease, Alzheimer's disease, and cancer. They hope to discover ways to encourage the action of the protective genes as well as to discourage the damage inherent in some genes' actions."

The implications are immense. "Should genetic engineering or genetic surgery ever become a reality, a physician would be able to adjust the DNA . . . to [its] original efficiency," says Georgakas. "Ultimately, the genetic code itself may be alterable. When this is possible, diseases based on genetic inheritance would become curable."

"In such a scenario, individuals whose cholesterol has risen to unacceptable levels might receive genes based on those enjoyed by [people with low cholesterol]," says Orlock. "Gene therapy also holds promise for treatment of declining immune function, as well as for heart disease, arthritis, diabetes, Alzheimer's disease, and Parkinson's disease."

And treating such diseases can lengthen life.

CLK-1

Biologist Siegfried Hekimi and his research colleagues at Montreal's McGill University have discovered a gene that Hekimi calls clk-1. This "clock" gene seems to affect the life cycle. In that regard, it fits into the theories of programmed death.

Hekimi has modified clk-1 in nematode worms so that the creatures live more than five times their normal span—although Hekimi notes that such worms are dull, lethargic, and passive, even for worms.

Humans don't seem to have clk-1, but we do have genes that are similar. If those genes could be modified so that humans could live six times longer, American life expectancy could theoretically be stretched from 76 years to nearly 400 years.

THE PROBLEM WITH ENGINEERING

Unfortunately, genetic engineering as a technique to help people live longer is many years away. Most of us will probably be dead before we will get the chance to benefit from it.

So although genetic engineering is a tantalizing prospect, the trick will be living long enough to take advantage of it.

TELOMERE THERAPY

Telomere therapy is based on the structure of DNA chromosomes. The telomere is the tip of a human chromosome.

Explains Medina in *The Clock of Ages*, "When a cell gets ready to divide, it first has to replicate all of its chromosomes . . . [but] the tip never gets replicated, and the new cell has fewer genetic sequences at its tip than the old cell."

Since, as Orlock puts it, "the essential units of DNA are safely ensconced toward the center of the chromosome," cutting off the ends doesn't cause much damage. But every time that the cell divides, it loses a little more of the chromosome.

"After a certain number of cell divisions, the telomere might be gone, and operating genes might be damaged," Moore writes in *Life Span*. "This self-induced amputation would eventually lead to a loss of essential genes," Medina says.

Since these genes govern (among other things) the body's ability to stay healthy, Orlock believes that losing them "could contribute to conditions such as atherosclerosis, osteoarthritis, osteoporosis, and diabetes."

What's more, the shortening of the telomere may cause the cell to reach the Hayflick limit. As Orlock says, "When the telomere becomes too short, the cell, like the last bearer of a family's name, dies without offspring."

But if science can find a way to lengthen the telomere, the cell can reproduce many times without losing essential genes. The body may be able to stay alive and healthy longer.

TELOMERASE

Cancer cells don't lose their telomeres. So they must have some way to prevent losing them—and they do. "Tumor cells prevent themselves from dying by manufacturing an enzyme called telomerase," Orlock says. Telomerase, explains Moore, allows the DNA to duplicate without losing its telomeres.

Telomerase appears not just in cancer cells but also in germ cells—"immortal" cells that produce the egg and sperm. Unfortunately, most of the body's other cells don't have telomerase. Consequently, nothing protects those cells from losing genes and starting to malfunction.

There may be hope. Orlock explains: "Offering [telomerase] to healthy cells might keep them alive. Thus cells essential to the functioning of our hearts, lungs, or brains could be kept from dying. Rather than cell lines dying out and their absence compromising the health of an organ, they could reproduce and keep a vital function going."

TELOMERE TROUBLES

It's a great theory, but it may not work.

First, says Kanungo in *Genes and Aging*, "Whether the shortening of telomeres is the cause or effect of aging is not known." And Moore asks, "Does [the telomere] play a central causal role in aging, or is it simply another entry in the catalogue of 200 known changes that occur in cell aging, some of which are significant, some of which are not?"

Hayflick says, "Biogerontologists are waiting anxiously for new developments as this fascinating story unfolds." And the rest of us will wait with them.

HORMONES

Hormones regulate body functions ranging from metabolism to reproduction to damage repair. "When an organism hatches or is born, its rate of growth, its sexual maturation, and the duration of its adult reproductive phases are *all* controlled by hormones," *Aging* explains.

So it makes sense that hormones may be central to aging and death.

HORMONE LOSS

One hormone theory starts from a simple fact: "After the age of 30, the levels of numerous hormones [in humans] begin to decline," Orlock says. "If medicine could maintain these hormones at near-normal levels, the consequences of weakened muscles, fragile bones, and diminished immune defenses might never arise." And people would live longer.

DEATH HORMONE

It sounds eerie, but there may actually be a hormone that kills its host. Its host is the body in which it lives.

"One hormone theory proposes that aging occurs when a certain hormone is produced by the pituitary gland," says DiGiovanna. "The hormone changes the functioning of cells so that biological aging occurs. Since the changes produced by the hormone ultimately result in death, this theory has been called the death hormone theory."

"The hormone," Hayflick says, "[is] formally known as [the] decreasing oxygen consumption hormone, or DECO." DECO may participate in the suicidal processes proposed in the genetic clock theories.

DECO can be fought, DiGiovanna says. "It is believed by some researchers that the production of this hormone, and therefore the processes of aging, can be slowed by restricting the amount of food that is eaten."

That is, if there is such a thing as DECO. According to *Search for Immortality*, "No one knows if DECO exists." Scientists are searching, but they haven't yet found this theoretical hormone.

THE ANTI-HORMONE VIEW

"Despite the profound effects that the [hormone] system has on our bodies, there is no direct evidence that it is the origin of all age changes," says Hayflick.

Besides, he says, many animals age and die, just like humans, but not all of them have the complex system of hormones that humans have. If hormones cause death, why do hormoneless animals die?

It's a question that remains unanswered. Until it gets answered, this theory remains unproven.

HUMAN GROWTH HORMONE

Growth hormone is a heavy hitter in keeping the body strong and healthy. Orlock calls it "the body's jack-of-all-trades, contributing to the healing of wounds and major repairs of skin, bone, and other assets that need upkeep every day. It also affects the strength of the immune system and the metabolism of fats."

But at some point in adulthood—the experts differ as to whether it's age 30, 50, 60, or another age— "the levels of human growth hormone sharply decline and in some older persons, production seems to shut down altogether," Mindell writes in *Earl Mindell's Anti-Aging Bible*. "As the level of growth hormone declines, so does body function." In other words, the body ages.

Logically, then, restoring human growth hormone should restore youth. And in fact, it may.

According to the American Geriatrics Society's guide, "studies of growth hormone suggest that it reverses some of the metabolic effects that are associated with aging."

In particular, a study completed in 1990 by Dr. Daniel Rudman of the Medical College of Wisconsin, which was published in the *New England Journal of Medicine*, disclosed that giving growth hormone to men over 60 reduced their amount of fat, increased their amount of muscle, and made their blood healthier. Orlock notes: "Elderly men saw the aging clock turn back twenty years; their 'middle-age spread' melted away, the fat composition of their bodies decreasing by an average of 14 percent. Meanwhile, their muscles grew by 9 percent. Their skin gained thickness; some bones began getting stronger. Even their livers and spleens grew to resemble the size of those organs in younger people, reversing the trend of shrinkage typical in old age." As health writer Stephen Rae described it in a *Men's Health* magazine article, "Supplementation . . . appeared to cancel ten to twenty years of some age-related changes."

Unfortunately, Rae goes on, "Researchers at the University of California at San Francisco reported . . . [that] human growth hormone supplements may also raise your risk of diabetes and . . . promote the growth of prostate cancers."

Still, growth hormone is an encouraging substance. More research needs to be done to find out for certain what it can and cannot do.

CAN YOU BUY GROWTH HORMONE?

Not easily.

Mindell say: "In the United States, the only medically accepted use of growth hormone is to supplement it in growing children with documented low levels. Growth hormone is available in many countries outside the United States, and many clinics abroad are dispensing the stuff with a free hand."

IT'S NO MIRACLE CURE

Not everyone is enthusiastic about growth hormone:

- "Giving supplemental growth hormone to the aging body will restore some lost muscle mass and redistribute your fat, but it will not affect many other common aging changes," Fossel says. You'll still age and die, he believes.

- Although everyone ages, not everyone seems to run low on growth hormone. So high levels of growth hormone may not prevent aging—which means that giving people extra growth hormone probably won't prevent it, either.

- Giving people growth hormone may bring on side effects such as arthritis, cancer, diabetes, and acromegaly (swelling of the head).

- Southern Illinois University School of Medicine physiologist and longevity scholar Andrzej Bartke said (in a *New York Times* article on long-lived mammals), "Prolonged treatment with large doses [of growth hormone] should be looked at very carefully for side effects, including shortening of life span."

Orlock adds, "These risks appear to be preventable by carefully calculating the dosage"—but, she adds, no one knows the dangers of using growth hormone over the long term.

There simply isn't enough information available about growth hormone to make a final decision about it. Like many theories, it still needs more testing.

But, writes Moore in *Life Span*, "Human growth hormone remains another of those promising leads in longevity research."

IMMUNITY

The immune system looks for foreign elements that don't belong in the body; when it finds them, it releases antibodies to attack them. If it fails, the body can get sick—and can even die.

"With age, the immune system's ability to produce antibodies in adequate numbers and of the proper sort declines," Hayflick says. For example, says *Aging: A Natural History*, "the flu that a young person shakes off after a day or so may be a serious threat to the very aged."

This decline in the immune system may be the very reason that everyone dies.

AGAINST THE THEORY

"The theory suffers from several flaws," says Hayflick. "First, it is not universal; some animals that age do not have a well-developed immune system." In other words, a malfunctioning immune system can't cause aging and death if creatures that don't have an immune system nevertheless age and die.

Besides, even in animals that do have immune systems, not all immune cells decline. *Aging: A Natural History* describes immune cells called macrophages that "show no impairments in function. On the contrary, during normal aging, and especially in people stricken by Alzheimer's disease, macrophages appear to become hyperactive in the brain."

So the immune system, although important to health, may not be central to the important problem of why we age and die.

BODY TEMPERATURE

Our body heat may be killing us.

According to *Aging on Hold*, "[There is] a feeling among scientists that a leading cause of genetic damage, and hence aging, is that we live internally at 98.6 degrees Fahrenheit." Exactly why is not yet clear.

But what if we lower the heat?

- Hayflick reports, "Surgical and chemical means have succeeded in turning down the thermostat in monkeys and rats." As a result, the animals suffer less genetic damage over time—Ronald Hart, Ph.D., of the National Institute on Aging says, "Cooling cuts DNA damage by 25 percent, all by itself"—and less DNA damage can lead to longer life.

- In humans, "[if] the body's thermostat could be lowered from two to three degrees Celsius, there would be no negative side effects, while life might be extended from twenty to thirty years," says Georgakas.

- According to *Search for Immortality*, "Lowering core temperatures from 98.6 degrees Fahrenheit to 95 degrees Fahrenheit—technically, to the point of hypothermia—could increase life expectancy to about 140 years, while researchers at Northwestern University have calculated that the human life span could be increased to 200 years by dropping body temperature a full seven degrees."

There is a problem in testing this theory and putting it into practice. As *Search for Immortality* points out, "Just how to induce a lower internal temperature . . . remains a bit of a puzzle."

Not that there aren't ideas floating around. "This lowering could be accomplished through drugs, genetic engineering, mechanical devices, or mind techniques," Georgakas believes.

But no one knows for certain which of these techniques will work, and proof through experimentation seems a long way off.

CRYONICS

Another version of using cold to extend life is simply to freeze people.

"This method involves the placing of a fresh corpse in a container and freezing it to the temperature of liquid nitrogen," Georgakas explains. "Its advocates hope that the process will preserve the body in a state of suspended animation until such time as the disease that killed the body can be reversed or until aging itself has become a curable disease."

There is a precedent for this hope. Reports *Search for Immortality*, "Studies of hibernating animals have shown that some frogs and turtles routinely survive for days or weeks with much of their bodies frozen solid. In the laboratory, scientists have succeeded in reviving hamsters after short periods in which portions of their body fluids apparently turned to ice."

At least thirty people have been frozen immediately after death. Orlock says, "While no one has ever been brought back from freezing, experiments with animals are keeping hopes for eventual revival, so to speak, alive."

DRAWBACKS

The flaws in cryonics are many. Freezing can kill cells. The only way to prevent the body's cells from dying is to insert what Hayflick calls a cryoprotective agent—an antifreeze—into the bloodstream. But since the blood will be frozen solid, Hayflick says, "the cryoprotective agent cannot penetrate into all cells. In the laboratory, this limits the amount of tissue that can be frozen and thawed, with most cells surviving [limited] to scraps no bigger than a matchstick head."

Freezing seems particularly dangerous for the body's most crucial component. Hayflick says, "When even tiny portions of animal brains are frozen and then thawed using the methods of the cryonicists, considerable cell destruction can be seen." There's no point in being thawed out if the process destroys your brain.

Moreover, reports *Search for Immortality*, "Most of the scientists sympathetic to the idea . . . believe that a reliable freezing and thawing process is unlikely to be perfected in the lifetime of anyone now living."

"Even its most optimistic supporters acknowledge that the present freezing technology may be so primitive that the chance of successful revival is exceedingly slim, a mere percentage of 1 percent," Georgakas says.

Cryonics may work someday, but that time seems far off.

CLONING AND ORGAN REPLACEMENT

Starfish can regrow chopped-off limbs. Can replacement parts be created for humans? When your heart ages and begins to fail, can you get a new one?

Search for Immortality quotes biologist Paul Segall, who suggests cloning human bodies—minus the brain—and using the body parts of the clones to replace injured or ailing parts in the bodies of sick or wounded people. Or doctors might transplant the brain of a sick person into a healthy clone of that person. If you can replace your body (or its parts), you can theoretically live as long as your brain holds out.

"That such a scenario could ever become possible is problematic," Georgakas warns. "The fact that [cloning and brain transplants] appear to be possible does not guarantee that they actually are possible."

MECHANICAL REPLACEMENTS

There is, theoretically, another source for body parts. "Today, science has provided pacemakers for tired hearts, plastic tubing for destroyed arteries, mechanical joints for worn-out bones, and transplants for dysfunctioning organs," Georgakas notes.

"While results thus far have been disappointing, work continues on developing artificial hearts, lungs, livers, and eyes, and even devices to substitute for failing portions of the brain," Orlock says.

Will it work? Will science ever be able to give you an artificial body that needs only an oil change and a 10,000-mile checkup?

No one knows, but it's intriguing to consider.

NANOTECHNOLOGY

Nanotechnology sounds like an opium dream. But it's rooted in scientific theory.

"K. Eric Drexler . . . a computer scientist who trained at the Massachusetts Institute of Technology . . . coined the term *nanotechnology* to describe [a] future generation of molecule-size machines so small that they would be measured in nanometers—tens of billionths of an inch," *Search for Immortality* explains.

Dr. Wesley Du Charme, in his book *Becoming Immortal: Nanotechnology, You, and the Demise of Death*, explains: "The essence of nanotechnology is control of matter at the molecular level, that is, the manipulation of molecules to build desired structures. The kind of engineering envisioned has structures being built molecule by molecule with complete positional control of each molecule so as to arrive at the desired structure."

Nanomachines might be able to repair or replace damaged brain cells and other microscopic body parts. They could keep diseased hearts going and aged nerves operating.

There's one obstacle to using nanotechnology to keep the body alive—it doesn't exist yet. "For the present," Orlock says, "the potential of building 'nanomachines' remains only theory."

IS THERE A SINGLE ANSWER?

PROBABLY NOT.

"None of the theories of aging are able to explain all of the changes observed in any organism," write Ricklefs and Finch in *Aging: A Natural History*. DiGiovanna agrees: "Each theory is supported by some evidence, and each can explain certain aspects of biological aging. However, none tells the complete story. This may be because aging results from a combination of causes."

It would be ideal if there were a single cause of aging, because that would mean that a single procedure—perhaps a yearly injection—could keep people alive indefinitely.

It may still turn out to be that way. But at the moment, no one knows the true causes of aging and death.

AFTERWORD

IT CAN BE DONE.

That sentiment formed in my head as I researched and wrote this book. Although several ideas mentioned here contradict each other, and others remain unconfirmed, many are clear and true—the benefits of diet, exercise, companionship, and stress management, for example. They indicate that living a long time is clearly within our grasp.

And it doesn't have to be a miserable life. That's another conclusion that I found. Living a long life doesn't have to mean spartan self-denial. Healthy foods can be tasty foods, sex and friendship are good for longevity, and some exercises can actually be fun. What a relief: a long life that you can actually enjoy while living it.

That's a third concept that came as I was writing. It's possible to live not just a long life, not just a long and healthy life, but a long, healthy, and happy life.

As a journalist, I'm a professional skeptic. Presented with a dream castle, I hunt for termites. The idea that health and happiness are inextricable parts of longevity seems too sweet for my usual acrid attitude. Every life has struggle and pain and fear, and any life can end at any time.

Yet the evidence stares back at me—and at you. If you're smart and lucky and determined, your life can last more than a century, much of it with a sound body and positive emotions. It sounds too good to be true . . .

But it *can* be done.

Advanced glycosylation endproducts (AGEs). Chemical compounds produced by glycation. AGEs can attach themselves to proteins and cause nearby molecules to cross-link with each other.

Alchemy. An early form of chemistry; one of its goals was to find a way to achieve long, youthful life.

Amino acids. Chemical compounds that are the building block of proteins.

Antioxidant. A substance that can prevent oxygen from damaging cells. See **free radical**.

Aspartame. An artificial sweetener, sold under the commercial name NutraSweet.

Beta carotene. A nutrient, found in orange-yellow fruits and vegetables and dark-green vegetables, that the body converts to vitamin A.

Biological age. The body's age according to its appearance, fitness, and ability to function.

Caloric restriction. Reducing food intake by at least 20 percent in order to achieve long life.

Calorie. A measurement of energy, specifically the amount of heat that can raise the temperature of one kilogram of water by one degree centigrade. In nutritional terms, a calorie is a measure of the amount of energy that the body absorbs when it metabolizes food.

Carbohydrates. Organic substances containing carbon, hydrogen, and oxygen, commonly found in plants and used by the body as sources of energy and nourishment.

Carotenoids. A family of natural pigments in fruits and vegetables. The human body uses them to produce vitamin A.

Catalase. An enzyme suspected of helping to slow down the aging process by protecting the cells against damage by free radicals.

Cholesterol. A fatty substance in the body that helps to form cellular walls. High levels of cholesterol have been linked to heart disease.

Chronological age. The actual age of a human body since birth.

Clinkers. Waste products that the body accumulates from interactions among cells.

Coenzyme Q-10. An antioxidant, found in cells, that helps deliver energy to the cells. It may also protect against life-threatening diseases.

Collagen. A fibrous protein that composes much of the body's connective tissues. Collagen cross-linking is suspected as a cause of aging.

Complex carbohydrates. The starchy parts of vegetables and grains, and a source of energy that the body can use more efficiently than fat or simple carbohydrates.

Cross-linking. The forming of bonds between molecules. Cross-linking of tissues can make the body less flexible, impair its functions, and possibly cause aging.

Cryonics. A technique of freezing a dead or dying body or a body part in the hope of reviving it at a later date.

Decreasing oxygen consumption hormone (DECO). A hormone suspected as a cause of aging.

Dehydroepiandrosterone (DHEA). A common hormone, produced less and less as the years go by, that is suspected of keeping the body youthful.

Endorphins. Hormones that produce sensations of relaxation and even euphoria. Laughter, sexual activity, and aerobic exercise can trigger the flow of endorphins.

Enzyme. A protein that helps to regulate and control chemical reactions in the body.

Error catastrophe. A theory in which the body's accumulation of damage causes aging and death.

Estrogen. A sex hormone, produced by the ovaries, that is suspected of fighting heart disease and triggering breast cancer.

Fat. A substance, solid at room temperature, in which the body stores unused energy.

Fiber. The indigestible parts of plants. Fiber is useful in preventing cancer and free radical damage.

Free radical. A molecule with an extra electron. Free radicals of oxygen can damage cells and cause many fatal diseases and conditions, especially heart disease.

Free weight. In strength training, a barbell, dumbbell, or other unattached heavy object that can strengthen muscles when lifted.

Fructose. The sugar in fruit.

Genetic program activation. A theory of aging in which the body's genes cause the body to age and die at a predetermined time or stimulus.

Gerontology. The scientific study of aging.

Gerovital. A supposed cure for aging, popular in the 1950s, that turned out to be little else but Novocain.

Gland. An organ that secretes substances such as hormones into the body.

Glutathione. An antioxidant compound, produced in the body, that fights cancer and heart disease.

Glycation. A process in which sugar binds to proteins in the body and impairs their function. Glycation may be a central cause of aging.

Grazing. Eating small amounts of food throughout the day as an alternative to the traditional three meals per day.

Growth hormone. See **human growth hormone**.

Hayflick limit. The maximum number of times that a cell can divide. Named for its discoverer, Dr. Leonard Hayflick, the Hayflick limit is central to theories of programmed death.

High-density lipoprotein (HDL). A form of cholesterol, known familiarly as "good" cholesterol, that removes cholesterol from tissues and thereby protects the body against heart disease.

Hormone. A substance that the body manufactures and secretes into the blood, and that alters cellular activity and regulates body function. Insulin, estrogen, and testosterone are examples of hormones.

Human growth hormone. A hormone secreted by the pituitary gland. Human growth hormone has been suspected of being a key to long biologically young life.

Insulin. A hormone that converts blood sugar into a form that the body's cells can use. Excess insulin can destroy arteries, raise levels of LDL cholesterol, and trigger diabetes.

International unit (IU). A pharmaceutical measurement of vitamins and other supplements.

Life expectancy. The potential length of a person's life based on the average for that person's group. The group can be defined by gender, nationality, race, or other factors.

Low-density lipoprotein (LDL). A form of cholesterol, known familiarly as "bad" cholesterol, that sticks to artery walls and can cause heart disease and other maladies.

Melatonin. A hormone involved in the cycle of sleeping and waking, sometimes suspected to aid in keeping the body young.

Metabolism. The body's chemical processes, especially those that apply to the use of energy.

Monounsaturated fat. A type of fat, found in olive oil, canola oil, and avocados, that may lower cholesterol levels and stabilize blood sugar levels.

Omega-3 fatty acids. A type of fat, found in fish, that may help to prevent heart and circulatory-system disease.

Osteoporosis. A potentially fatal condition that causes weakening of the bones.

Phytochemicals. Substances in plants that, when eaten, can fight off cancer, heart disease, and other ailments. The best known phytochemicals are the antioxidants.

Polyunsaturated fat. A type of fat, found in processed foods and some cooking oils, that can promote cancer, artery disease, and immune-system problems.

Progesterone. A hormone produced in the ovaries that may help to fight uterine cancer.

Progestin. A synthetic hormone used with estrogen to ameliorate estrogen's harmful effects.

Programmed death. A theory of aging in which the human body is thought to start destroying itself at a particular point in its life.

Progressive relaxation. A form of stress reduction that involves relaxing muscle groups in succession.

Protease inhibitors. A group of phytochemicals, found in beans and seeds, that fight cancer.

Protein. An organic compound made of amino acids and used throughout the body. Protein, which is in the cells of animals and plants, is essential to the diet, although excessive amounts can be dangerous.

Recommended Daily Allowance. Values that the U.S. Food and Drug Administration has placed on nutrients, defining the amount of each nutrient a body needs each day.

Recommended Dietary Allowance. Values that the Food and Nutrition Board of the National Academy of Sciences has placed on nutrients, defining the amount of each nutrient a body needs to maintain good health.

Relaxation response. The condition of being physically relaxed, brought about by meditation or prayer.

Resistance machine. A device that uses stacks of weights to help an exerciser build strength.

Saccharin. An artificial sweetener that may promote cancer.

Saturated fat. A type of fat, found in meats, dairy products, and fried foods, that is believed to promote cancer.

Simple carbohydrates. Carbohydrates better known as sugars. Simple carbohydrates can build fat, which can promote many life-threatening ailments and conditions.

Sodium nitrite. A preservative and flavor enhancer, found in processed meats, that can promote cancer.

Somatic mutation. A theory in which the accumulation of genetic mutations in cells is said to cause aging and death.

Sucrose. A simple carbohydrate best known as white table sugar.

Sun protection factor (SPF). A measurement of the power of sunscreen to prevent skin damage.

Superoxide dismutase (SOD). An antioxidant enzyme, found in long-lived species, that may promote longevity.

Telomerase. An enzyme that prevents the shortening of telomeres during cell reproduction. It allows cells to reproduce without losing any of their genes and thus may be a key to keeping cells healthy and organisms long-lived.

Telomere. The tip of a DNA strand. After the reproduction of some cells, the telomere of the daughter cell is shorter than that of the parent cell. After several reproductions, the telomere may be cut off entirely, exposing the strand's crucial genetic information to being cut off itself during subsequent reproductions.

Testosterone. A sex hormone produced in the testicles that can build muscle and bone, and promote cancer.

Transcendental meditation. A relaxation technique in which the meditator focuses on a word until he or she is no longer stressed by the outside world.

Trans fat. Hardened polyunsaturated fat, found in cakes, potato chips, poultry, beef, and fried foods, that can promote heart disease and cancer.

Triglyceride. A molecule containing fat, used to transport fat in the blood and to store it.

Ultraviolet. The type of solar radiation that causes skin cancer and other skin damage.

Vitamin. An organic substance, found in food, that can help to regulate the body's metabolism.

BIBLIOGRAPHY

Age Erasers for Women: Actions You Can Take Right Now to Look Younger and Feel Great. Emmaus, Pa.: Rodale Press, Inc., 1994.

Arnot, Robert, M.D. *Dr. Bob Arnot's Guide to Turning Back the Clock.* Boston: Little, Brown, 1995.

Aronne, Louis J., M.D., with Fred Graver. *Weigh Less, Live Longer.* New York: John Wiley & Sons, Inc., 1996.

Barnard, Neil, M.D. *Eat Right, Live Longer: Using the Natural Power of Foods to Age-Proof Your Body.* New York: Harmony Books, 1995.

Bellamy, Denis. *Ageing: A Biomedical Perspective.* Chichester, West Sussex, England: John Wiley & Sons Ltd., 1995.

Bortz, Walter M. II, M.D. *Dare to Be 100.* New York: Fireside Books, 1996.

Carper, Jean. *Stop Aging Now!* New York: HarperCollins, 1995.

Chopra, Deepak, M.D. *Ageless Body, Timeless Mind: The Quantum Alternative to Growing Old.* New York: Harmony Books, 1993.

Crews, Douglas E., and Ralph M. Garruto, eds. *Biological Anthropology and Aging: Perspectives on Human Variation over the Life Span.* New York: Oxford University Press, 1994.

Deeb, Richard G., D.N. *Live to Be 100+: Healthy Choices for Maximizing Your Life.* San Francisco: Robert D. Reed Publishers, 1995.

DiGiovanna, Augustine Gaspar. *Human Aging: Biological Perspectives.* New York: McGraw-Hill, Inc., 1994.

Dilman, Vladimir M. *Development, Aging, and Disease: A New Rationale for an Intervention Strategy.* Translated and edited by John K. Young. Switzerland: Harwood Academic Publishers. Originally published in Russian as *Four Models of Medicine.* Leningrad: Meditsina Publishers, 1994.

Dollemore, Doug, Mark Giuliucci, and the editors of *Men's Health* magazine. *Age Erasers for Men: Hundreds of Fast and Easy Ways to Beat the Years.* Emmaus, Pa.: Rodale Press, Inc., 1994.

Du Charme, Wesley M., M.D. *Becoming Immortal: Nanotechnology, You, and the Demise of Death.* Evergreen, Colo.: Blue Creek Ventures, 1995.

Ford, Norman D. *18 Natural Ways to Look and Feel Half Your Age.* New Canaan, Conn.: Keats Publishing, Inc., 1996.

Fossel, Michael, Ph.D., M.D. *Reversing Human Aging.* New York: William Morrow, 1996.

Fries, James F., M.D. *Living Well: Taking Care of Your Health in the Middle and Later Years.* Reading, Mass.: Addison-Wesley, 1994.

Georgakas, Dan. *The Methuselah Factors.* Chicago: Academy Chicago Publishers, 1995.

Griffith, H. Winter, M.D. *Complete Guide to Symptoms, Illness & Surgery for People Over 50.* New York: The Body Press/Perigree Books, 1992.

Hayflick, Leonard, Ph.D. *How and Why We Age.* New York: Ballantine Books, 1994.

Kanungo, M.S. *Genes and Aging.* Cambridge, England: Cambridge University Press, 1994.

Klatz, Ronald, M.D., and Robert Goldman, M.D. *Stopping the Clock: Why Many of Us Will Live Past 100—And Enjoy Every Minute!* New Canaan, Conn.: Keats Publishing, 1996.

Kotulak, Ronald, and Peter Gorner. *Aging on Hold: Secrets of Living Younger Longer.* Orlando, Fla.: Tribune Publishing, 1992.

Live Longer, Live Better. Pleasantville, N.Y.: The Reader's Digest Association, Inc., 1995.

Medina, John J. *The Clock of Ages: Why We Age—How We Age—Winding Back the Clock.* Cambridge, England: Cambridge University Press, 1996.

Mindell, Earl, R.Ph., Ph.D. *Earl Mindell's Anti-Aging Bible*. New York: Fireside Books, 1996.

Monte, Tom, and the editors of *Prevention* magazine. *Staying Young: How to Prevent, Slow, or Reverse More Than 60 Signs of Aging*. Emmaus, Pa.: Rodale Press, 1994.

Moore, Thomas J. *Lifespan: Who Lives Longer—and Why*. New York: Simon & Schuster, 1993.

Orlock, Carol. *The End of Aging: How Medical Science is Changing Our Concept of Old Age*. New York: Birch Lane Press/Carol Publishing Group, 1995.

Ricklefs, Robert E., and Caleb E. Finch. *Aging: A Natural History*. New York: Scientific American Library, 1995.

Ryback, David, Ph.D. *Look Ten Years Younger, Live Ten Years Longer: A Man's Guide*. Englewood Cliffs, N.J.: Prentice-Hall, 1995.

Search for Immortality. Alexandria, Va.: Time-Life Books, 1992.

Walford, Roy, M.D. and Lisa Walford. *The Anti-Aging Plan: Strategies and Recipes for Extending Your Healthy Years of Life*. New York: Four Walls Eight Windows, 1994.

Williams, Mark E., M.D. *The American Geriatrics Society's Complete Guide to Aging & Health*. New York: Harmony Books, 1995.

Willix, Robert D., Jr., M.D. *Healthy at 100: 7 Steps to a Century of Great Health*. Boca Raton, Fla.: Shot Tower Books, Inc., 1994.

INDEX

A

Accumulation
  theories of, 273-278
    accumulation of mutations,
      274-275
    error accumulation, 273-274
    error catastrophe theory,
      273-274
    glycation and collagen
      cross-linking, 275-276
    somatic mutations, 274-275
    waste product theories, 277
    wear and tear, 278
Activities, finding exercises in
  everyday, 152-153
Additives, food, 56-60
Aging, no single answer to, 293
Aging process, stopping or
  delaying, 273-278
Antioxidants, 51-53
Aspirin, 266-268

B

Beta carotene, 236-238
Biologically young bodies, 14
Bodies, building healthy, 14-17
Body temperature, 289-290
Born, how one is, 13
Bowman-Birk inhibitors, 50
Breakfast, 103-104
Breathing, 151-152

C

CAD (coronary artery disease),
  216
Caffeine, 87-89
  controversies, 87-88
  and longevity, 88
  moderation, 88-89
Calcium, 70-72
  and bones, 70
  consuming more calcium, 71
Calisthenics, 143-144
  chin-ups, 144
  push-ups, 144
  sit-ups, 144
Calories, 31-32
Carbohydrates, 39-42
Catalase, 261-262
Cholesterol, 45-49
CLK-1, 282
Cloning, 291-292
Coenzyme Q-10, 263-264
Collagen cross-linking, 275-276
Contact with others, 190-198
  communities, 196-198
    nursing homes, 197-198
    old folks' homes, 196-198
    retirement communities,
      196-197
  family life, 194
  living with loved ones, 191-195
  marriage, 191-194
    happy, 193-194
    lengthening of life, 192-193
  pets, 195

Control
  beyond human, 7-13
    changing rules, 10-11
    genetic factors, 11-12
    how one is born, 13
    killer genes, 9-10
    living longer, 13
    longevity genes, 9
    race, 12-13
    sex, 11-12
  of one's life, 167-171
COPDs (chronic obstructive
    pulmonary diseases), 217
Cryonics, 290-291

D

Death
  hormone, 285
  statistics, 3-4
  theories of programmed,
    279-281
DHEA (dehydroepiandrosterone),
    258-259
Dietary supplements, 231-252
Drinking, 184-186
Drugs, 264-269
  aspirin, 266-268
    consulting a physician, 268
    dangers, 267
    dosage, 267
    stroke controversy, 267-268
    those needing, 266
  checking, 265-266
  doing without, 268-269

E

Eat
  foods to, 89-94
  number of meals to, 102-103
Education, and intelligence, 22-24
Estrogen, 81-83, 254-257
Exercises
  aerobic, 126-138
    exercises, cycling, 135-136
    and free radicals, 129
    high-impact and low-impact
      aerobics, 137
    miscellaneous exercises, 137
    running, 132-133
    swimming, 134-135
    walking, 130-132
    weight-bearing exercises, 127
    workings of aerobics, 127-129
    workouts, 130
  beyond boundaries, 150-153
    nonexercise exercises,
      151-153
    T'ai Chi, 151
  case against, 112-113
  case for, 113-115
  getting started, 120-122
    getting checkups, 120-121
    getting partners, 121
    going slow, 122-123
    having fun, 121
    having goals, 121-122
    writing down comments, 122
  miscellaneous, 150-153
  myths, legends, and lies,
    115-119
    exercise can kill, 119
    exercise wipes out bad foods,
      118

exercising when old, 115-116
gym needed for proper
    workout, 118
no pain, no gain approach,
    116-117
not needing exercise earlier
    in life, 118
risks of injures, 117
resistance machine exercises,
    146-147
schedules, 123-126
    elapsed time after eating, 124
    minimum and optimum, 123
    regularity, 124
    varying workouts, 126
    warm-up, cool-down,
        125-126
    weeks or months to exercise?,
        124-125
and sleep, 184
specific, 126-154
sports, 153-154
strength
    calisthenics, 143-144
    curls, 145
    exercises, 143-147
    free-weight exercises, 145
    lateral raise, 146
    presses, 145-146
    training with equipment, 145
strength building, 138-143
    benefits of strength, 138
    disadvantages and dangers,
        139
    gyms, 142
    health clubs, 142
    into the future, 143
    partners, 143
    trainers, 142

workout advice, 139-141
stretching and flexibility,
    147-150
    how to stretch, 147-148
    specific stretches, 148-149
    yoga, 149-150
to live long, 111

F

Family life, 194
Fat, 32-39
Fiber, 54-56
Foods
    additives, 56-60
        avoiding contaminants, 60
        bacteria, 59
        contaminants, 59-60
        pollutants, 59-60
        salt, 60
        sodium nitrite, 60-61
        sweeteners, 57-58
    best to eat, 89-94
    buying, cooking, and eating,
        95-107
        baking food, 105-106
        broiling food, 106
        caloric restriction, 98-101
        food preparation, 104-107
        frying food, 106-107
        meals, 101-104
        organic produce, 95
        raw food, 104-105
        steaming food, 105
        vegetarianism, 95-98
    hormones in, 80-87
        estrogen, 81-83
        insulin, 85-87

progesterone, 83
testosterone, 83-85
power of, 29-30
to avoid, 89-94
to eat, 89-94
Foods, contents of, 31-89
calories, 31-32
carbohydrates, 39-42
complex carbohydrates,
39-40
simple carbohydrates, 41-42
cholesterol, 45-49
cutting, 47-49
disclaiming power of, 46-47
good, 49
power of, 46
fat, 32-39
big picture, 38-39
monounsaturated fat, 37
omega-3 fatty acids, 37-38
polyunsaturated fat, 35
saturated fat, 33-35
trans fats, 35-36
triglycerides, 36-37
fiber, 54-56
minerals, 69-79
boron, 69-70
calcium, 70-72
chromium, 72
iron, 73-74
magnesium, 74
potassium, 75
selenium, 75-77
sodium, 77-79
zinc, 79
phytochemicals, 50-54
proteins, 42-45
consuming too much, 43-44
muscle controversy, 44-45

need for more, 44
protein-rich foods, 42-43
quantity need, 42
vitamins, 61-69
A and carotenoids, 61-63
B_1, 64
B_2, 64
B_3, 65
B_6, 65
B_{12}, 65-66
B, 63-66
biotin, 67
C, 67
D, 67-68
E, 68
folic acid, 66-67
K, 69
Free radicals, stopping the, 52-53

G

Genes
killer, 9-10
longevity, 9
Genetic clock theory, 280-281
Genetic engineering, 281-283
Genetic program activation,
280-281
Glands and hormones, 252-261
dehydroepiandrosterone
(DHEA), 258-259
estrogen, 254-257
benefits, 254-255
estrogen plus progestin,
256-257
plus progesterone, 256
risking use, 255-256
risks, 255

women at risk, 257
melatonin, 260-261
Glutathione, 53-54, 262-263
Glycation, 275-276
Growth hormone, human,
  286-288

H

HDLs (high-density lipoproteins),
  9, 49, 67, 81, 84
Heart disease, 216-217
Hormones, 285-286
  in food, 80-87
  and glands, 252-261
  human growth, 286-288
  loss of, 285
  miscellaneous, 87
Human growth hormone, 286-288
Humans, beyond control by, 7-13
  changing rules, 10-11
  genetic factors, 11-12
  how one is born, 13
  killer genes, 9-10
  living longer, 13
  longevity genes, 9
  race, 12-13
  sex, 11-12

I

Immunity, 288-289
Injures, risks of, 117
Insulin, 85-87
Intelligence and education, 22-24
Iron, 97

L

LDLs (low-density lipoproteins),
  9, 49, 67, 70, 81, 132
Life
  control of one's, 167-171
    getting, 168
    income, 168-170
    learning, 171
  one should lead, 24-25
Lifespan, maximum, 507
Liquids; *See* Drinking
Live, time people expect to, 3
Living
  locations, 199-215
  longer, 13
Locations, living, 199-215
  Caucasus, 203-205
  climate, 208
  Ecuador, 206-207
  fountains of youth, 199-200
  geographical factors, 208-213
  Hunza, 207-208
  Japan, 200-203
  Okinawa, 202-203
  Pakistan, 207-208
  polluted places, 214-215
  rural versus urban, 214
  sunlight, 209-213
    bright side of sun, 210-211
    clothing, 213
    medical cautions, 213
    sunblock, 211-212
    sunscreen, 211-212
    sunshine allotment, 211
    tanning without sun, 213
  temperature, 208-209
  United States, 205-206
  Vilcabamba, 206-207
Lung diseases, miscellaneous, 217

M

Marriage, 191-194
Maximum lifespan, 5-7
Meals, 101-104
Medications; *See also* Drugs
    and supplements, 227-269
        and ancient days, 229
        Bogomoletz's serum, 230
        Gerovital, 230
        and today, 231
Meditation, 159-160
Megadoses, 250-252
Melatonin, 260-261
Mind, 17-24
    attributes, 17-19
    choosing right, 17-24
    and emotions, 18-19
    and intelligence and education,
      22-24
    and stress, 20-22
    training the, 157-167
      meditation, 159-160
      optimism, 157-158
      relaxation, 158-167
      stress reduction, 158-167
Minerals, 245-249

N

Nanotechnology, 292-293
Nitrite, sodium, 60-61
Nursing homes, 197-198

O

Occupations, 173-175
Omega-3 fatty acids, 37-38, 264
Organ replacement, 291-292
OSHA (Occupational Safety and
    Health Administration), 175

P

Pets, 195
Phytochemicals, 50-54
    antioxidants, 51-53
    glutathione, 53-54
    protease inhibitors, 50
Polluted places, 214-215
Progesterone, 83, 256
Progestin, estrogen plus, 256-257
Protease inhibitors, 50
Protein, 42-45, 97

R

Race, 12-13
RDAs (Recommended Daily
    Allowances), 234-235
Relaxing, 186
Retirement, 175-177
    communities, 196-197

S

Salt, 60
Sex, 11-12, 188-190
    celibacy conundrum, 189
    legends, 189-190
    statistics, 188-189

SHBG (sex hormone binding globulin), 81
Sleep, 178-187
  amount needed, 179-180
  benefits of, 179
  effects of sleeplessness, 179
  exceptions, 180
  in later years, 181
  schedules for, 182-186
    afternoon napping, 183
    awakening early, 183
    drinking, 184-186
    exercising, 184
    fretting, 184
    getting to sleep, 187
    getting up at a regular time, 182
    late dining, 184
    relaxing, 186
    tranquilizers, 186
    when to go to sleep, 187
  what it does, 179-181
Sleeping room, 181-182
Smoking, 215-225
  at second hand, 225
  defense, 218-221
    antioxidant defense, 220
    being doomed, 220-221
    geezer defense, 219-220
    quitting smoking and regaining health, 221
    relaxation defense, 219
    slimness defense, 218-219
    smog is worse defense, 219
  effects, 216-218
    cancer, 217
    heart disease, 216-217
    miscellaneous effects, 218
    miscellaneous lung diseases, 217

kills, 215
  quitting, 222-224
    quit date, 222
    on quit day, 223
    relapses, 224
    withdrawal symptoms, 223-224
SOD (superoxide dismutase), 261-262
Sodium, 77-79
Sodium nitrite, 60-61
SPF (sun protection factor), 211-212
Sports, 153-154
Statistics, death, 3-4
Strength exercises, specific, 143-147
Stress, 20-22
Stroke controversy, 267-268
Substances, miscellaneous, 261-264
  catalase, 261-262
  coenzyme Q-10, 263-264
  glutathione, 262-263
  omega-3 fatty acids, 264
  superoxide dismutase (SOD), 261-262
Supplements
  B_2 (niacin), 238
  B_6 (pyridoxine), 238-239
  B_{12} (cobalamin), 239
  B vitamins, 238-239
  beta carotene, 236-238
  dietary, 231-252
    megadoses, 250-252
    multivitamin and multimineral supplements, 250
    negative side, 233-234
    positive side, 232-233

Recommended Daily
  Allowances (RDAs),
  234-235
  so what should one do?, 234
  specific supplements, 245-249
folic acid (folate or folacin), 239
and medications, 227-269
  ancient days, 229
  Bogomoletz's serum, 230
  Gerovital, 230
  and today, 231
minerals, 245-249
  calcium, 246-247
  chromium, 247
  iron, 247
  magnesium, 248
  potassium, 248
  selenium, 249
  zinc, 249
miscellaneous B vitamins, 239
vitamin A, 235-236
vitamin C, 240-242
  cautions, 241-242
  dosage, 241
  what supplements can do,
    240-241
vitamin D, 242-243
vitamin E, 243-245
vitamins, 235-245
Sweeteners, 57-58
  artificial sweeteners, 58
  safer sweeteners, 58
  sugar, 58

T

Telomerase, 284
Telomere theory, 283-284
Temperature, body, 289-290
Testosterone, 83-85
Theories, miscellaneous, 281-293
  body temperature, 289-290
  cloning, 291-292
  cryonics, 290-291
  genetic engineering, 281-283
    CLK-1, 282
    problem with, 282-283
  hormones, 285-286
  human growth hormone,
    286-288
  immunity, 288-289
  nanotechnology, 292-293
  organ replacement, 291-292
  telomere theory, 283-284
Tranquilizers, 186
Triglycerides, 36-37

V

Vegan, 100 percent, 97-98
Vegetarianism, 95-98
  100 percent vegan, 97-98
  iron, 97
  limitations and variety, 96-97
  protein, 97
  versus illness, 95-96
  vitamin B_{12}, 97
  zinc, 97
Vitamins, 61-69, 97

W

Waste product theories, 277
Wear and tear, 278
Weight
    ideal, 15-17
    stable, 16-17
Work, 172-177
    challenging or congenial?,
      172-177
    occupations, 173-175
      jobs don't cause longevity,
        174
      long-living people get good
        jobs, 174
      workplaces, 174-175
    retirement, 175-177

Y

Youth, fountains of, 199-200

Z

Zinc, 97